GOING MAD?

Understanding Mental Illness

GOING MAD?

Understanding Mental Illness

Michael Corry and Áine Tubridy

Newleaf

Published by
Newleaf
an imprint of
Gill & Macmillan Ltd
Hume Avenue, Park West
Dublin 12
with associated companies throughout the world
www.gillmacmillan.ie

© Michael Corry and Áine Tubridy 2001
0 7171 3283 8

Design by Caroline Moloney
Print origination in Ireland by redbarn publishing
Printed by ColourBooks Ltd, Dublin

This book is typeset in Garamond 10.5 on 12 point

The paper used in this book is made from the wood pulp of managed forests. For every tree felled, at least one tree is planted, thereby renewing natural resources.

A CIP catalogue record for this book is available from
the British Library.

1 3 5 4 2

Dedicated to all those who are experiencing soul pain and searching for solutions

It is a luxury to be understood
Ralph Waldo Emerson

CONTENTS

PROLOGUE — A NOTE FROM THE AUTHORS

<u>Keynote:</u> The Reason Why

Madness is as much a part of being human as is joy. It happens — it has its place — yet it makes us recoil in fear. To go mad is considered a fate worse than death, yet paradoxically it holds an awesome fascination for us. Like the scene of a road traffic accident, madness compels us to slow down and take a look.

What has more stigma than madness? If you have 'it', you become one of society's undesirables and as such find yourself alienated and mistrusted. History tells a pitiful tale when it comes to the treatment of the mad. They were related to as an ethnic group and as such were 'cleansed'. Have times changed?

We see madness as understandable. It has a logical history embedded within its own unique context. If all the contributing factors were fully appreciated, madness would emerge as inevitable. If any of us were 'in their shoes', the outcome is likely to be the same. For us, madness is no longer a case of a rogue gene going bump in the night — it is a reflection of the difficult business of living and experiencing life.

Madness is best seen as an event occurring along the spectrum of sanity-insanity. Unconsciously we all suspect that given the right climate, any of us could find ourselves on the other side of the divide, i.e. that no-one is immune to madness.

Madness is:
- being constantly afraid that something harmful is about to happen to you, about which you can do nothing
- feeling pleasure only when you consume mood-altering substances
- wilfully harming another human being to obtain a sense of satisfaction, pleasure or power
- being so filled with self-loathing that you mutilate yourself, withhold food, or end your life
- thinking thoughts and feeling compelled to behave in ways you don't wish to, and being unable to stop them
- feeling that you are trapped in a life lacking joy with no meaning

- losing contact with everyday reality and having beliefs that are not shared by others

As clinicians voyaging through the world of psychological distress, we noticed that our findings failed to match the territory so categorically mapped out by mainstream thinking. While the official map may have been technically correct in terms of symptoms, signs and classification, it fell far short of capturing the unique origins of madness, its idiosyncratic mental and emotional content, not to mention the soul pain — the crisis of spirit. *Middle-aged mother of four, suffering from endogenous depression with suicidal ideation* seemed a thousand miles away from what was really going on inside this client. What we were witnessing on a daily basis forced us to go beyond the domain of traditional explanations and search for answers elsewhere.

Trained as doctors in the science of medicine, we felt that we were cooking the books by ignoring what was patently not working. The established treatment methodologies were very hit and miss and were unreliable clinically. Medication could not be seen as curative because the people receiving it were becoming institutionalised chronic patients who spent years in hospital. If this were happening in any other branch of medicine and an audit was carried out, serious basic questions would be asked, such as: 'Has the right diagnosis been made?' and 'Are these patients on the right treatment regime?' — if the answers were 'no' there would be a public outcry.

Working at the coalface we found it hard to comprehend the different standards for our population. It seemed to be acceptable to be treated for depression for years and still to be depressed! To be treated for schizophrenia for an entire lifetime and still be psychotic! In addition, the side effects of the medication were frequently worse than the so-called disease.

Our quest for knowledge has introduced us to the cutting edge of psychotherapy, philosophy, anthropology, sociology, mind-brain chemistry, quantum physics and bioenergy. The spiritual dimension now seemed impossible to ignore. Had we been satisfied with the answers offered in our medical training, life would have been much easier. It was a surprise to discover such huge gaps in a science we had so completely trusted. 'First do no harm', the tenet enshrined in the Hippocratic oath, did not seem to apply in the area of psychological distress. To make matters worse, nobody seemed to mind and the indifference to asking new questions and introducing change was shocking.

In collecting data for this book, I (Michael Corry) found documents from 1981–2 which were written in response to the horrors of long-stay institutional care as it was commonly practised in Ireland. The following quote gives a sense of how these experiences were beginning to impact personally on me.

'I was stunned and changed by what I witnessed in the back wards of St Brendan's hospital. The conditions were repulsive. The impact of seeing hundreds of unkempt human beings of all ages lying, sitting and walking in smelly, shabby hallways and corridors, looking like inmates of a concentration camp, was staggering. This human zoo was caused by diffusion of authority, lack of accountability, lack of interest, conceptual gaps, the culture of silence, the inappropriateness of the medical model, involuntary detention and pure staff laziness. This was the undeniable barometer, the true measurement of care, love, respect and civil liberties.'

We have learned that seeing ourselves as spiritual beings having a human experience not only opens the door to the widest possible canvas, but invites in the exquisite uniqueness of each one of us on our own soul journey. Notwithstanding similarities and differences with respect to race, colour, creed, gender, socioeconomics or family of origin, the existence of a soul dimension puts our individuality beyond question — no two souls are alike.

Practising from this position is like chalk and cheese, night and day, flat earth and round earth. It gives room to draw on unlimited resources in the interest of healing and to place psychological distress of any kind within a larger framework. In this way psychiatry takes on its true meaning, that of 'soul-healing' (*psyche* meaning 'soul' and *iatriea* meaning 'healing').

We see this book as a liberation text, which will empower the psychologically distressed and those close to them by helping to normalise and make sense of their predicaments. We hope this book will encourage people to relate to 'madness' not as a disease or a mistake, but rather as a messenger whose mission is to draw attention to a lack of balance in the way a person might be living. This turns their symptom into a critical aspect of themselves to be explored, expanded upon and used with a view to transforming their own lives. In contrast to squeezing psychological distress into an orthodox pathological framework, it creates more room for the qualities of hope, expansiveness, diversity and interconnectedness. In our view, this is the contemporary meaning of alchemy.

It appears to us that the first step on the road to personal growth and freedom has to do with compassion. The love of the self (which comes with a peaceful and calm feeling) is too often eclipsed by conditioning, deprivation, abuse, fear and self-loathing. From the moment of conception onwards our beings soak up everything around them like sponges; the good, the bad and the ugly. Many of us can find the burden too much and experience a soul pain of such proportions that our mind-body-spirit organism can't take it any more and wants out. Suicide, like madness (or indeed any human act) has its own unique implicit rationale. To fail to embrace this universal truth is to turn back the evolutionary clock, where the notion of self-consciousness, free will, love and soul-purpose is not even on the horizon.

Forgiveness and acceptance are the travelling companions of compassion. They merge to create heart energy and the consciousness of softness, where there is no place for shame, guilt or atonement.

Mary Oliver's poem 'Wild Geese' calls out to us with the theme of personal liberation, both through the awareness of the 'soft animal' and a reminder that we have a place in the grand scheme of things.

WILD GEESE

YOU DO NOT HAVE TO BE GOOD.
YOU DO NOT HAVE TO WALK ON YOUR KNEES
FOR A HUNDRED MILES THROUGH THE DESERT, REPENTING.
YOU ONLY HAVE TO LET THE SOFT ANIMAL OF YOUR BODY
LOVE WHAT IT LOVES.

TELL ME ABOUT DESPAIR, YOURS, AND I WILL TELL YOU MINE.
MEANWHILE THE WORLD GOES ON.
MEANWHILE THE SUN AND THE CLEAR PEBBLES OF THE RAIN
ARE MOVING ACROSS THE LANDSCAPES,
OVER THE PRAIRIES AND THE DEEP TREES,
THE MOUNTAINS AND THE RIVERS.
MEANWHILE THE WILD GEESE, HIGH IN THE CLEAN BLUE AIR,
ARE HEADING HOME AGAIN.

WHOEVER YOU ARE, NO MATTER HOW LONELY,
THE WORLD OFFERS ITSELF TO YOUR IMAGINATION,
CALLS TO YOU LIKE THE WILD GEESE, HARSH AND EXCITING...
OVER AND OVER ANNOUNCING YOUR PLACE
IN THE FAMILY OF THINGS.

MARY OLIVER

INTRODUCTION

Keynote: Mental Spin Cycles

'Miss, do you want that toasted?'

The sandwich vendor's voice gives Mary a jolt. It's as if he's speaking to her from a different planet.

'No, I'm in a hurry,' she snaps. 'Give it to me as it is.'

Mary has started feeling sick. *'What's taking him so long,'* she thinks, exasperated. *'I'm going to lose it if I don't get out of here.'*

'Are you all right?' asks the voice.

'I'm fine, just a bit too warm.' *'Oh God,'* thinks Mary, *'here we go again. . .'*

Sweat breaks out on Mary's body. Her knees are shaking, the room is spinning, her stomach begins to heave. Pins and needles spread across her face and hands, her mouth clams up, suddenly she can't say what she wants to say. She feels removed from what is actually happening, not fully present, as though she is a spectator watching herself order lunch.

'Why is my heart racing?' she thinks. *'Has anyone noticed my hands shaking? If I don't get out of here right now I'll do something stupid. I'll lose my mind and wake up in three months' time in some loony bin. What's happening to me? I must be going mad!'*

How does the average person explain a strange experience like the one above? How has ordering a sandwich, something a five-year-old could do, turned into a terrifying ordeal? Mary has been going to the same sandwich bar on her lunch break for years. Why has it suddenly become a frightening place?

One of the most alarming experiences has to be losing control over one's thoughts, feelings and behaviour. People know instinctively that if they lose control of the command post, they are no longer running the show.

Where does Mary go to make sense of these seemingly illogical experiences? Like most people, she hopes and prays that they will eventually pass and there will be no need to mention them to anybody. What would people think? She can hardly mention it to her boss and colleagues without fear of judgement, nor to her family without fear of worrying them. She could mention it to her doctor but is afraid of what his diagnosis might be. Early schizophrenia? Manic depression? Brain tumour? Whatever it is, it doesn't look good.

If, weeks later, there has been no improvement and Mary goes to her doctor, the most likely outcome is that he will diagnose stress, anxiety or depression and prescribe something 'for the nerves' such as Xanax or Prozac.

Six months later Mary is no better. She has taken a number of sick days, avoids the sandwich bar altogether, goes into the supermarket and bank only when they are empty and is short tempered with those around her. She has been back to her doctor a number of times. He has increased the dosage and has added in another medication. To complicate matters, Mary's concentration is noticeably worse. She is forgetful and finds it increasingly difficult to cope with the demands of work. She is afraid she is going to lose her job. She is thinking, 'I'm certainly not the same girl that won the karaoke competition at last year's Christmas party.'

Since she is on all the right medication but still feels no better, Mary starts to believe that there must be something seriously wrong with her mind. She relays these fears to her doctor who suggests a consultation with a psychiatrist. To Mary this is the final nail in the coffin. All her worst fears have been confirmed.

Mary runs the video in her mind. Years of medication. In and out of psychiatric institutions. Obviously she loses her job. Obviously her boyfriend leaves her. Clearly her friends will not want to know her and her family will only tolerate her out of pity. Poor old Mary. Of course nobody will be surprised — sure wasn't Aunt Kitty on pills and seeing a psychiatrist for years? Didn't she spend endless months in institutions? Don't they say that madness runs in the family?

Mary's situation differs dramatically from someone receiving a diagnosis of diabetes, peptic ulcer, angina or arthritis. The mind in all these states will remain 'intact'. People suffering from these diseases can still socialise, do their jobs and generally live a 'normal' life while their body heals. They don't have to deal with the terrifying experience of losing control of their thinking, that all-important rudder by which they steer their lives.

Everyone knows that when you have a physical problem you get lots of sympathy and support. We have all heard the heroic stories of fund-raising activities for sick children needing urgent operations. There is no danger of being stigmatised and shunned. But whoever heard of a sponsored walk for 'Johnny the schizophrenic', who needs a safe space and hours of specialised one-to-one and group therapy? Psychiatric problems are not dinner party conversations. You can eat out on your last chiropractic consultation or cataract operation, but not on your last panic attack or suicidal thought.

Psychological distress has a stigma that physical disease doesn't share. This adds an extra layer of difficulty over and above the symptoms themselves. Well-meaning suggestions are laced with judgements and advice. They imply that with enough 'willpower' and 'backbone' it is possible to summon up the necessary strength to overcome the problem. Those who can't quickly pull themselves together are thought to be spineless, weak, unco-operative and lazy — in a culture where success and achievement are venerated, who wants to be any of these? No wonder people like Mary want to keep their problems to themselves. Shame and secrecy become travelling companions. Jobs, promotions and relationships are at stake. After all, who can trust someone who has had a 'nervous breakdown'?

The fear of going mad (like Mary) is not exclusive to high levels of anxiety and panic, although it is the commonest source. There are many other weird symptoms which terrify people simply because they have no way of explaining them, nor have they ever met anyone else who has had similar experiences.

The phenomenon of flashbacks associated with a traumatic event is a case in point. Imagine having a meal with colleagues in the cafeteria at work, when following a sudden noise you find yourself instantly catapulted back into reliving the entire traumatic experience of a recent near-fatal road accident. While it is happening you may cry out, shake, sweat and grip the table as if it were the car's steering wheel. Wild-eyed and terrified, you may find yourself pushing past 'bystanders' to rescue your child who had been thrown through the windscreen.

Who would blame you or others for thinking that you were going mad, given such unexpected and off-the-wall behaviour? It is not uncommon for survivors of trauma to vividly re-experience the smell of burning, blood or smoke in ordinary present time situations, not to mention the sound of breaking glass, screeching tyres, explosions etc. Lacking a framework of explanation for such extra-ordinary experiences, most people would question their sanity and become extremely fearful.

Unexpected psychic and paranormal experiences happen to many of us, yet when they occur they can cause great fear. Spiritual 'openings' — for example, those arising out of a 'born again' charismatic conversion — can be accompanied by dramatic phenomena such as seeing lights, hearing celestial music, speaking in tongues, seeing angels, becoming infused with bliss and love and feeling inexplicably drawn to connect with others. It is also not uncommon in grief to feel the presence of a dead loved one or even to see them, but when this happens it can be deeply disturbing.

How do you interpret an 'out-of-body experience' in which you found yourself looking down on your body as it was going through a car crash, a resuscitation, an operation or a rape? It is scary stuff when you don't understand what is going on in your own mind and when you are afraid to talk about it. Likewise, people need explanations for other psychic experiences such as seeing auras, picking up the emotions of others, intuiting future events, etc.

These experiences are difficult to share because of the fear of being thought strange. In days gone by the place to bring stories like these would have been to the shaman, the medicine man or wise elder who would have made sense of them within an accepted cultural framework. In their absence these experiences may end up in a doctor's consulting room, running the risk of being related to as 'psychiatric' or 'pathological'.

Through the increased use of recreational drugs, in particular those that have hallucinogenic properties, a wide range of altered states are happening to more and more people. Some of these psychedelic experiences, where the consciousness of the self changes and expands, can be blissful and meaningful; but others can be terrifying and cause high levels of anxiety, once again producing the fear of insanity.

In our work as therapists, many of our consultations are with the Marys of this world, as well as those who experience flashbacks, spiritual openings, psychic and paranormal phenomena and drug-induced hallucinations. What all these people have in common is the fear that they are on the verge of 'losing' their minds, their identities, their sense of who they are and how to manage their lives. If that happens, who is in charge?

If my mind is the place which my memories call 'home' and if I have lost it, then where am I to be found? Who will re-mind me when I awake that the person sleeping next to me is my partner, that the children running into the bedroom are my own, that I am expected at work in an hour's time, that I still have my head cold and that my mother is coming for dinner tonight? Who will re-mind me that if I don't pay the phone bill soon I will get cut off, that I must drive on the correct side of the road, turn up at my place of work and return to my own home at the end of the day? If my mind takes care of all this and I lose it, then am I going to end up like a zombie, a mindless body being shepherded from the chair to the bed? Or will I be dragged away by the police and the men in white coats for attempting to direct traffic half-naked on the high street?

This book is our attempt to answer these questions in plain language, by charting the course of psychological distress from the minor to the major, clearly documenting what happens and what doesn't. We aim to make even madness understandable and inseparable from the experience of being human.

SECTION 1

CHAPTER 1 — FEAR

Keynote: Our Most Basic Instinct

The mind is a place which of itself can make a heaven of hell, or a hell of heaven. Milton

Fear can drive us mad. Fear is the engine behind our need to be a success, to be thought well of, to look good and to belong. It also drives anxiety, panic, depression, grief, worry, paranoia, obsessions and compulsions, mania, schizophrenia and other distressing psychological experiences. Its key role in creating physical dis-ease is now well established. Peace of mind, contentment and trust are often absent in the years leading up to a diagnosis of high blood pressure, heart attacks, peptic ulcers, migraine and even cancer.

Wave a wand, take away fear and you could empty the psychiatric hospitals and put the pharmaceutical companies out of business. So what is this fear? What is it doing in our lives? How does it work and what can be done about it?

Every emotion has a function. In the case of fear it is to alert us to the presence of any potential threats in our environment. These can be small or large, ranging from being afraid you will be late to fearing that your breast lump will turn out to be malignant. On a daily basis we operate on a continuum between fear and safety, constantly making the necessary adjustments to keep ourselves up the safety end where there is peace of mind. The essence of fear is summed up in the statement: *something that means a great deal to me is being threatened and I know I can't protect it.* Fear says 'pay attention and get ready'. It demands vigilance, prompting us to mount a response as soon as we find evidence that all is not well.

Rescue comes in the form of the fight-flight response, a primitive survival reflex which has evolved to keep us safe. This response is activated and operational before we have time to think about it. We don't hang about in front of a charging lion or a speeding car. We are no longer cavemen but we still live in a jungle, the urban jungle, where the lion is the taxman and the car an approaching deadline. The things we fear have changed, but the fight-flight response is still the same, just sitting there and waiting to be triggered.

Meet the Adrenaline Molecule

In the Introduction, Mary is standing at the sandwich bar — in the grip of a pounding heart, a cold sweat and the desire to bolt for the door — running high levels of adrenaline. This is the cause of her panic attack. For some weeks she has been worried about losing her job because the company is downsizing. If this happens, what will people think? How will it look to her family and friends? They might think that Mary can't do anything right, isn't she always screwing up?

Mary can't stop running mental images of how people would gossip about her in the dreaded scenario of losing her job. She feels oversensitive, exposed and more self-conscious than usual, imagining that people are looking at her. Queuing makes her feel trapped and unsafe. Even the thought that it is time to get a sandwich starts Mary's adrenaline rising.

Once in the bloodstream, molecules of any chemical can influence how we think, feel and behave. Take alcohol for example. As the blood levels rise our body relaxes, a feeling of mellowness grows, worries of the past and concerns for the future fall away, our confidence increases and we connect more easily with others. The more alcohol consumed the more changes that occur, but not all are pleasant. When one is drunk, the alcohol molecule has taken over the control tower and is now running the show. When we are drunk we drive cars dangerously, argue with people, can be overly amorous, maudlin or melancholy. On the other hand we might become funny and entertaining, or fall asleep. A chemical shift has taken place and now we see the world through 'beer goggles'. The effects are dose- and thought-related, ranging from a warm glow to rancour.

Unlike alcohol, adrenaline molecules — the chemicals of fear — are not taken by the glass but are generated by us internally through the 'movies' in our minds. From Mary's first inkling of insecurity in the queue, her adrenaline rose. This chemical shift accounted for all her symptoms. She is in the grip of the fight-flight response. Fighting or making a quick getaway is the only move; and since there is nothing tangible to fight, she takes flight.

Staying Alive

The fight-flight response was vital for the physical survival of the caveman. He lived in a world where he was both hunter and hunted; a tasty morsel on the food chain. Outside the safe-ty of his cave, he had to be vigilant all the time, constantly scan-ning his environment both for food and predators. Within a millisecond of perceiving danger the chemical cascade underly-ing the response instantly occurred. This caused the mental and physical changes he needed in order to render him capable of either fighting or fleeing. The choice depended on the magni-tude of the danger. His voice of experience would tell him, 'If I can't fight my way out of this one, I'll run.'

For either option the caveman needs the adrenaline to change his mind-body so that it has laser-sharp clarity and the brain speed necessary to work through a list of strategies. Sight and hearing is enhanced to bring in more information. His focus of concentration is entirely on the emergency. His muscles become more active. Facilitating this is the combination of increased heart rate and faster breathing. He sweats more to prevent overheating. Like an Olympic sprinter about to race, he has been transformed into a finely tuned, high-performance organism.

For most of us, on a daily basis, the rush of adrenaline is usually generated not by a charging wild animal or the sound of a starting gun but by *internal images of threat*. Individuals differ about what threatens them. If I'm not fazed by being unpunctual, then a traffic delay won't bother me. If on the other hand I feel that my life depends on being on time, then a traf-fic jam will make me tense, anxious and panicky.

Ironically, unlike the caveman who can discharge this built-up energy, the executive in the urban jungle is generally not in a position to flee from his car or attack the one in front. Consequently he sits it out awash with chemicals that have no outlet, or else he succumbs to road rage. We are all familiar with the experience of our thoughts nudging us in and out of the adrenaline state, sometimes many times a day. This same mechanism is what awakens us from a nightmare, terrified and gasping for breath with a racing heart, tense muscles and sweaty wet sheets.

Adrenaline-driven thoughts morning, noon and night without let-up can 'lift' us to another level of defence, where we cross a line and enter the world of madness, the place where thought loses contact with reality. In the practice of psy-chiatry this shift is labelled mania, schizophrenia or psychosis. The vast range of symptoms which characterise these states, while called a 'chemical imbalance', are actually the extreme end of the fight-flight spectrum — a last ditch effort to survive, to escape a threat-filled world. In this altered state of consciousness, our defence becomes purely mental. We see ourselves as all-powerful and therefore safe, or else the victims of a well-orchestrated conspiracy where vigilance and paranoia pay off.

WHERE IS THE LEMON OR THE ORGY?

Imagine yourself in your kitchen picking up a fresh lemon and with a sharp knife cutting it in two. Look at the glistening juicy surface and the lemony smell. Now visualise cutting a segment and sucking it. You may notice a bitter taste in your mouth as your facial muscles grimace, saliva forms and you want to swallow. No *real* lemon was involved in the process, but the same physiological responses occurred as if there had been. Something invisible, a thought, has been made real. Scientists could take a sample of the saliva produced, examine its properties and quantify it. They would, however, have no success in locating the presence of a lemon in the brain. The image in the invisible realm has resulted in the formation of chemical molecules which exist on the physical plane. Mind into matter.

Where would sex be without anticipation, fantasy and lustful images? Physical arousal can occur even in the absence of an actual sexual partner, for example, during masturbation when the source of the stimulation is entirely in the mind. You can have fun at an orgy without being physically present. Who has not experienced an erotic dream? Once again molecules, this time sexual hormones, are created by our mental movies.

The Fear Cascade

Awakening to the sound of breaking glass downstairs in the middle of the night, your instant conclusion is that an intruder is present. Alarmed, your heart begins to pound. With tense muscles, short of breath and covered in a cold sweat, your racing mind looks at possible scenarios. In terror, you shake your partner awake explaining in urgent whispers, 'There's a burglar downstairs.' A calm voice informs you that they forgot to put the cat out. Phew! This eminently safer scenario brings about an instant physiological reversal of all your symptoms. Feeling calmer, you are asleep in five minutes.

If we see a thought as an impulse of energy and information which, like a TV remote control, has the potential to change our channels, we can understand how we are the creators of our own chemical responses. There are thoughts behind the molecules associated with sadness, joy, fear, anger and other emotional states. The unique image world of each one of us is inseparable from our emotional states. In the same way that a car's movement depends on the driver's planned journey and the presence of fuel.

THREATS TO OUR IDENTITY

In the modern jungle, while physical threats can occasionally occur, most of them are created by our mental imagery and our need to defend our beliefs, particularly those relating to our social identity. If I know myself as a person who has high standards, is successful, hardworking, honest, a good citizen and in control, then any challenge to these familiar ways of defining myself will make me feel threatened. Like the cavemen, we fall back on the fight-flight response in order to protect our status quo. Keeping our identity the same makes us feel secure.

Imagine a young child who is being abused or bullied. How they see themselves now changes radically. The identity they were familiar with vanishes. Now perhaps for the first time, they begin to feel vulnerable and useless, lose confidence and blame themselves. The world to them is no longer a safe place and they run fearful images of potential danger.

In many ways our caveman had less difficulty dealing with his threats, since they were largely external and explicit and he knew who his adversary was. Our threats are now both internal and external and operate at a much more subtle level. At times we may be unaware that we ourselves trigger the fear response by being self-critical and feeling that we are not being the people we 'should' be.

Constantly fighting the clock, or looking over our shoulder in case someone is taking advantage of us, we may not realise that these 'threats' are totally contrived by the way we see things, which may differ from the way they actually are. In subtle ways we are scaring ourselves.

Planet Earth — Are the Natives Friendly?

Looking at the earth as a spaceship and the population as its crew, you would not want to board it. Incredible conflict exists around the distribution of resources, politics and religion, race and gender. Environmental abuse is rampant and everywhere you look are the casualties of war, famine, institutional and sexual abuse, mass indoctrination, Coca-Cola consciousness, competition, power struggles and personal unhappiness. Humanity is in distress.

You cannot live on Planet Earth without experiencing a sense of threat. We must satisfy basic requirements, from our need for food and shelter to maintaining our self-image. We battle with deadlines, standards and goals. We are forced to learn how to delegate responsibility, share power and become team players in order to survive. The need to form relationships leaves us open to fears of rejection, abandonment, loneliness and betrayal of trust. The act of living in community with all our individual differences poses challenges when others disapprove of us and we cannot get our needs met. Speaking your truth, declaring your needs is not always a safe option. We may find ourselves harshly judged. The fear that our dreams will not come true and the dis-illusionment when they don't is with us daily. Some of us can feel desolate, with an overwhelming sense of meaninglessness and futility.

As spiritual beings, the human experience for which we have signed up can seem a daunting task. Many of us feel profoundly alienated, with no manual or instruction book for being human. Some of us would prefer not be here because we find the world so toxic and hostile. Those of us who sense that the angelic realm is our true home can feel desolate at such remoteness from our origins, stranded in a harsh place where we must be ever-vigilant of the inhabitants.

We believe that people who experience altered states such as schizophrenia have reached the point where they find it extremely difficult to commit themselves to being fully present on the earth plane. They have created, under pressure — much like the endorphins of marathon runners — the specific chemistry to 'trip out' and leave this reality. They have succeeded in manufacturing their own hallucinogens. As such they behave in a way that resonates with ET wanting to get off the planet. Once 'out there' under the influence of their own mind-altering substances, they may neither be able to return nor want to.

For these individuals, psychosis or going 'mad' is the only available solution to the dilemma of having to deal with prolonged threat — it is more viable than suicide. The necessary skills to bring control over the situation may be lacking and literally running away might not be an option. This may particularly hold true for the young and vulnerable. From within their mindset their move makes perfect sense, albeit bewildering to an onlooker.

Symptom as Messenger

If we see symptoms as expressions of an underlying personal history, they can be valuable sources of information — they can point the way to a solution. In much the same way as a pain in our big toe draws our attention to an ingrown toenail, a psychological symptom alerts us to an underlying problem. Anaesthetising the symptom or shooting the messenger defeats its purpose and is not a wise move.

Imagine pasting over the flashing oil light on the dashboard of your car. Doing so is perilous, because now the need for lubrication goes unheeded and unmet. Yet we regularly find the symptoms of fear obliterated, medicated out of existence before the underlying cause has been explored.

CHAPTER 2 — SELF-LOATHING

Keynote: Love's Executioner

> 'I'd better get going or I'll be late for work.'
> 'I'd never forgive myself if I missed her birthday.'
> 'Thank God I wore this dress, I look great.'
> 'I can't believe I was so stupid.'
> 'I deserve a medal for pulling that one off!'
> 'I must have been out of my mind.'
> 'I think I made a great impression.'
> 'That's the last time I'll let that happen to me!'

These are the kinds of running commentaries that continue in everybody's minds on a daily basis. What they imply is that we are a divided self. One part, our 'observer', is looking at the other part, our 'performer' and making a judgement on the appropriateness of its behaviour. Good, bad, or indifferent.

How does our observer know what to think? The answer is, it is learned. From the very moment we are born, we find ourselves on the stage of life, subject to the gaze and observations of others. Whether we are a boy or a girl, wanted or unwanted, we are judged and adjectives are used to describe us. 'Isn't she a beautiful baby?' 'What a pity he cries so much.'

We learn our name by the fact that it is used when people address us. The same applies to the learning of words for things, like 'mummy' or 'daddy', 'bottle' and 'teddy'. How we see ourselves in our early years depends on what we are called by others and how we are seen in their eyes. If we are continually told 'You're no good, you're no good, you're no good,' we will inevitably internalise that information and repeat the mantra to ourselves, 'I'm no good, I'm no good, I'm no good.' The opposite is also true. This is how our internal conversations, both negative and positive, develop. Surely one of the fundamental laws of consciousness must be: *As I am perceived by others, so shall I perceive myself.*

A human being is a form of life that is self-conscious — that can see itself. It has the capacity to love or hate itself, to die naturally or kill itself. How we observe and assess ourselves dictates how happy and contented we feel. We can be our own best friend or our worst enemy. If we are at peace within ourselves then we can be at peace with those around us. The same applies with love.

In our practice there is nothing sadder than sitting opposite a fellow human being who loathes themselves one hundred per cent. Their observer, who ideally should be a loving friend and supporter, is pitted against them — a brutal oppressor. Their observer acts as love's executioner. It is as if part of the person is squeezing out the life-force and putting out the light.

This intrapersonal state is unsustainable. Many sufferers have either made or contemplated a serious suicide attempt — they are so full of hate for themselves. 'I just can't take it any more. I don't want to be here.'

It is not only parents, but also the critical eye of others, which trains our observer and shapes our view of ourselves. Every culture is awash with expectations, ideals, standards, rules, dictates and laws. If we fail to live up to these we can find ourselves disapproved of and on the 'wrong' list. As a child, we may find ourselves ridiculed and bullied for being too fat, too tall, too quiet, too bright, unpopular or ugly. In adult life we can find ourselves equally victimised, judged and stigmatised. (Stigma: a distinguishing mark of social disgrace.)

Our observer forms its opinion of us in other ways too. It pays attention to how worthwhile, valued and lovable we seem to be. As a baby we are profoundly affected by whether or not we are kissed, cuddled and attended to when we cry or get distressed. (Even in intrauterine life we are exposed to the thoughts and emotional chemistry of our mother, not to mention her ingested substances such as alcohol and nicotine.) The priming starts early.

If we are exposed to battering, sexual abuse, abandonment or neglect, our immature mind tries to make sense of it. It comes to the only conclusion it can, namely that *it could only be happening because we are bad*. We reason that nobody could love a bad child. Many years on, those people who had traumatic childhoods may firmly believe that they must have been responsible, that they somehow brought it on themselves.

Many adults, in spite of being adopted as babies into warm loving homes, become pilgrims searching for their biological parents; not only to establish roots but also to clarify doubts. They want to know the exact circumstances, the reasons why they were 'given away'. Many are plagued by self-doubt and loathing, for many years hearing the voice of their observer: 'If my mother had loved me she'd have kept me. What was wrong with me?'

As we grow into adult life the emotions of guilt and shame become attached to a myriad of rules, implicit and explicit.

Whenever we break one we inevitably feel guilty or ashamed. These feelings become the currency with which we pay for other people's disapproval. Families, friends, schools, employers, religions and governments can shape our behaviour by manipulatively triggering our guilt. Countless millions of young men were shamed into going to war and died. If we do not abide by the rules and be seen to live within the 'norm', we are stigmatised — another stick with which to beat ourselves.

The stigma and self-loathing that goes with psychological distress can sometimes be the worst part of the problem. Just look at the distinctions that are made between physical and mental dis-ease. Who can like themselves if they are seen by others as a non-coper, weak-willed, unreliable and not in control of their own mind? Mary, from the sandwich bar, sees herself in this light and hates herself for it. To make matters worse, the fear of being found out only serves to escalate her already high levels of fear.

Many suffering from psychological distress, if their self-loathing is intense enough, will begin a regime of self-punishment and destruction. They sentence themselves to a life of self-abuse which can take the form of exposing themselves to unnecessary danger, substance misuse, self-mutilation, rigorous dietary regimes, excessive physical workouts and suicidal behaviour. Their life is a reflection of the absence of any sense of personal worth. The mind at war with itself does a better job of inflicting maximum pain and is more of a threat to itself than any outside agent.

The imprint left by years of self-loathing is not likely to be shifted by a pill or a potion. It is one of the major causes of suicide — medication and hospitalisation do not appear to prevent it. Psychotherapy (*psyche* meaning 'soul' and *therapiea* meaning 'attendance') is the key healing intervention in self-loathing. Obviously the earlier it starts the more effective it can be. To this end *we would like to see self-loathing regarded as a clinical state* and named as such. Years and years of conditioning have to be peeled back and deconstructed. Their origins have to be made explicit before the old hardwired programmes can be released. The task of bringing an adult mind back to childhood emotions, and the false interpretations they engendered, is a science. However, insight alone is not enough. Now self-loathing sufferers have to learn to have self-loving thoughts and behaviours for the first time. In this process support is critical.

The act of bringing the 'observer' and the 'performer' together, unifying them in terms of their intention and sense of purpose, brings about a state of inner peace, love and *oneness with oneself*. We see psychotherapy as an applied philosophy, a way of life, not just a tool belonging to the clinical domain. With an understanding of the mechanism by which our inner world is constructed, we can make informed choices, actively seek out what we need and journey in the direction of integration and wholeness. This is the true meaning of personal liberation, beautifully sculpted in the following poem.

LOVE AFTER LOVE

THE TIME WILL COME
WHEN WITH ELATION,
YOU WILL GREET YOURSELF ARRIVING
AT YOUR OWN DOOR, IN YOUR OWN MIRROR,
AND EACH WILL SMILE AT THE OTHER'S WELCOME,
AND SAY, SIT HERE. EAT.
YOU WILL LOVE AGAIN
THE STRANGER WHO WAS YOURSELF.
GIVE WINE. GIVE BREAD. GIVE BACK YOUR HEART
TO ITSELF, TO THE STRANGER WHO HAS LOVED YOU
ALL YOUR LIFE, WHOM YOU IGNORED
FOR ANOTHER, WHO KNOWS YOU BY HEART,

TAKE DOWN THE LOVE LETTERS FROM THE BOOKSHELF,
THE PHOTOGRAPHS, THE DESPERATE NOTES,
PEEL YOUR OWN IMAGE FROM THE MIRROR.
SIT. FEAST ON YOUR LIFE.

DEREK WALCOTT

CHAPTER 3 — I DON'T WANT TO BE HERE

Keynote: The Bridge to Madness

'**O**uch!' I shout, **hopping around** the kitchen nursing my burnt hand. 'Quick, the cold tap. Aaahh, that feels better already. Now where is the burn cream?'

With a noxious agent that is physical, our instinctive response is to withdraw so that the pain connection is broken and we are safe again. Do you have toothache? Get to the dentist fast!

It is just as well we're designed so that these aches and pains alert us to physical threats and underlying disease. They warn us and give us the time to take protective action. Far from ignoring them, we respect and heed these mechanisms as messengers. But in the mental and emotional world we have a different relationship to warning signs. Fear, unless there is a physical external source like a burglar or a fire, is a nuisance, has no value and we want to get rid of it quickly. While the same holds true of the toothache which is both unacceptable and a nuisance, we drug the pain away at our peril. On goes the infection and we suffer more in the long run.

As a culture we have learned to dis-regard, compartmentalise and get rid of certain 'undesirable' emotions. Fear is at the top of the list. If we display it or admit to feeling it we automatically attract ridicule, disapproval and mockery. We can find ourselves described as 'not up to it', 'weak', having 'lost our nerve' and in macho organisations 'not one to be trusted'. In psychological jargon we are neurotic, inadequate and viewed as a non-coper. Medically we are labelled as suffering from anxiety, a panic disorder, or some class of phobia. The overall view of fear is that if you 'have it' you are lacking in something and, at worst, have a disease.

The upshot is that if we experience fear, particularly with no external source, we try to disown it and keep it a secret. Who wants to be stigmatised? If those around us view fear-full people as essentially no good, we will by implication also see ourselves as such. With fear and self-loathing now on board, life becomes intolerable and we start constructing a 'survival kit' to make life more bearable.

Within the fight-flight equation, since we can't fight or control our adrenaline level, or keep escaping to a safe place, we take the only option open to us — eliminate the enemy (fear) by putting it to sleep and anaesthetising it. Mary calls her fear 'the monster' and has spent months trying to tiptoe around it using various avoidance strategies such as bringing in a packed lunch, going into the supermarket only when it's nearly empty and boarding uncrowded commuter transport to and from work.

She has discovered that if she has a couple of drinks before going to a social gathering, she can keep her fear at bay and doesn't feel so bad about herself. She starts having a drink in the morning before going to work 'to settle the nerves' and brings a small bottle of vodka in her bag to keep the alcohol levels up and her fear levels down. She hates herself all the more for this new habit. Her problem is now compounded, she feels guilty and ashamed and her self-loathing escalates further. She frequently says to herself, 'If I could wave a wand, I'd be out of here.'

Life on Planet Earth is fraught with difficulties. It is at times dangerous, sad, depressing, empty, frustrating, stressful and boring. From time immemorial a range of survival kits have been devised. Ancient Rome created a world of distraction. Its population was captivated by reports of its wars and entertained by exotic games and an excess of wine, food and sex. In modern times the rat race mentality offers us a better, more fulfilled existence if we are educated, rich and surrounded by the right trophies and toys. What is the difference between an alcoholic and a workaholic; a re-creational drug and retail therapy; going to a rock concert and an evangelical rally? They all have the same goal — give me another reality! Anaesthetise this one — I don't want to be here! Doctors find themselves targeted to provide prescription drugs with this very aim in mind but in a socially validated and respectable way.

What do the states of depression, mania and schizophrenia have in common? They are an effort, an attempt, an unconscious coping strategy to deal with an immediate or a protracted series of difficulties. They are the signposts and the flashing lights; symptoms of unmet needs, of not fitting into a current life situation and of less than adequate resources. In this way, these states create a way of physically 'being here', while mentally and emotionally inhabiting another less distressing reality.

If we see psychological symptoms as an attempt to put right an overwhelming experience, pressure or stress, the result of a trip switch reaction, then conditions like schizophrenia and mania can be viewed as necessary and understandable. Now, there is method in madness. Seen in this light, there is no form of expression within the repertoire of 'what it is to be human' that does not make sense.

The current paradigm shift in consciousness has moved us to the position where, if we so choose, we can see ourselves as spiritual beings having human experiences rather than human beings having the occasional spiritual experience.

Within this framework, those who experience altered states of consciousness such as schizophrenia (splitting from current consensus reality) can be seen as individuals who have not, through fear, fully committed their spirit to the mind-body experience of being in the world. For them it is not a safe, user-friendly or open-hearted place. Their fragile sense of self, I-ness, or personal identity makes them excessively sensitive to the rough and tumble of the childhood years. They take in more of the world, becoming overloaded and easily overwhelmed. With an open boundary, what is on the outside becomes too easily what is on the inside. Feeling vulnerable and exposed, they retreat into the safety of their inner world, through the doors of a vivid imagination. Escaping into fantasy provides a hiding place.

These children learn to move between the inner and outer worlds of fantasy and reality. They have a foothold in each camp. This protective mechanism makes their lives more manageable. Years of withdrawing whenever they feel hurt leads them to connect less and less with others, preferring their own company and often engaging in solitary pursuits. Consequently, the sense of belonging to their peer group fails to develop and with time becomes less of a priority. At some point, usually in adolescence or early adulthood, when life presents them with a hurt or a challenge that is too much to bear, they withdraw totally into their inner world. At this point a line is crossed. 'I don't want to be here' has translated into a psychotic or schizophrenic break. Being human has become too tough. Now totally immersed in their inner world, it acts as the launching pad which intellectually, chemically and energetically propels them into the spiritual dimension.

This happens to John when he is nineteen. Although he's been able to survive within the relative safety of his school and fantasy world, John finds himself unable to cope with the commercial reality of his first job, which he finds terrifying. Having to concentrate, stay focussed, be sociable and meet deadlines are beyond his capabilities. Feeling increasingly inadequate and boxed-in, he is unable to fall back on the customary excuses used successfully in the past whenever he felt pressurised. 'Mum, I've a pain in my tummy and I'll only feel sick if I go to school.' 'I'm not playing with the kids on the road anymore because Tommy will call me names.' 'I don't want to go to the party because I'll only have to dance and I'll feel stupid.' 'I don't want any dinner, I'd prefer to stay in my room.'

So intense is John's fear and sense of alienation, he decides that in order to survive his only course of action is to withdraw.

He starts taking sick days and because he is on probation and seen by his boss as socially awkward and not up to speed with his work, he is fired. Now at home, he has time to inhabit his fantasy world more and more, finding solace and peace there. He experiences his parents' concerns and efforts to engage him as intrusive. To pacify them and justify spending more time in his room, he pretends to be composing CVs and searching out vocational options on the net. Spending days on end spinning in the vortex of his fantasy world he eventually gets sucked in and blown out into the world of boundlessness, oneness and God consciousness. Feeling reconnected to his spiritual origins, he feels 'at home'. We will join John later.

Unlike John, Julian finds a different way of avoiding being here. To the sound of polite applause he takes his seat in the spotlight in front of the Steinway grand piano. This is the moment he has been building up to for the last eight months and before that, for all his life.

His mother, a piano teacher, groomed Julian from the age of five to take the stage in the National Concert Hall. Not for him games on the road with neighbouring kids. He would routinely practice for four hours a day. The bookshelves groaned under the weight of the trophies he had won over the years — expectations of him soared. International success was a foregone conclusion. That is until last year when to the astonishment and disappointment of all, Julian returned suddenly from Paris, backing out of a prestigious scholarship at the Conservatoire after only two weeks. His mother was devastated and Julian knew she hadn't quite swallowed his excuse about being homesick.

Even though he tried to push it out of his mind, Julian couldn't forget the feeling of inadequacy in the presence of Europe's most promising young pianists. He realised from day one that he would not be the top of the class, or even close. Unaccustomed to being second best, confused, shocked and out of his depth, he packed his bags.

Back home, plans for his career continued but he found himself passed over for radio concerts and recordings by peers who in his view were less talented. Bitter now, his confidence plummets. Disillusioned and ashamed of the Paris debacle, he socially withdraws and rather than teach piano like his mother, he stops playing altogether. Frantic, his family contact his old mentor, who uses his influence to arrange a performance in the National Concert Hall. Julian jumps at the opportunity, particularly since the chosen piece is 'The Ascension' by Messiaen, the famous French mystical composer. 'How synchronous,' thinks Julian. 'Here is the opportunity to recreate myself.'

He begins a punishing practice regime, locking himself away for hours on end. He eats, sleeps and breathes Messiaen. He wants this performance to be flawless. Worried about making mistakes, he practices late into the night and unable to shut his mind down his sleep suffers. He talks obsessively about the performance and how it will launch him onto the international stage. He acquires an agent, instructing him to book a European tour and to arrange maximum publicity. He is encouraged by the success of the rehearsals and exhilarated by his plans, making him full of energy which further depletes his sleep.

As silence fills the hall on the special night, Julian feels an unexpected surge of power. After playing the first few bars he finds himself emotionally connected to each note. Inspired and 'at one' with the audience he senses that he is giving them the performance of a lifetime. Playing with such ease he feels he is channelling from the heavens. As he continues to play he feels as if he is floating above the piano, believing himself to be the Archangel Gabriel. He leaves the stage elated, feeling that his moment of triumph has finally come. Backstage he announces to everyone, 'You're looking at the greatest concert pianist of all time.'

Julian's manic 'escape' ensured that he didn't have to be here to deal with the painful reality of being ordinary, with its inherent possibility of failure. This was not part of his conditioned mindset. He was not going to be on the planet as a failure. Instead he created, through his rigid belief system, the energy and the chemistry of an altered state in which he inhabited his ideal persona. How this fitted in with others is another story and will be told later.

CHAPTER 4 — MORE THAN MEETS THE EYE

<u>Keynote:</u> The Heart of the Matter

Most of us looking at Mary in the sandwich bar would not be aware of her stressed-out thoughts. We would not hear her inner voice screaming *'I've got to get out of here now!'* Neither would we feel her heart racing and her rising levels of adrenaline pushing her into panic. All this information is invisible to our ordinary senses. Yet it is this very information that underpins all psychological distress and makes madness understandable.

Similarly, if a mobile phone rang no-one would be able to see or hear the electromagnetic waves which are transformed within the phone into a conversation. Certainly no-one would imagine that the radio playing in the background actually contains a tiny rock band. Mary, in her office that morning, didn't see or hear a postman delivering e-mails inside her computer. In the age of technology we take for granted that there is far more invisible than visible. We know that with imaginative and creative powers of thought anything is possible. Science fiction also points us in that direction.

Let us return to the human body and consider its layers of invisibility. Every second we are bombarded by incoming information which is given to us in manageable bite-sized pieces by our specifically designed sense organs. They filter out vast amounts of information such as light and sound waves which are irrelevant to our survival. Without this protective mechanism the hardware of our body would overload and crash.

If we take a look at what goes on inside the body it can be seen as the body electric — the city that never sleeps. Its trillions of cells all intercommunicate and depend on each other according to a brilliantly orchestrated electromagnetic master plan, certainly not one of human design. Every bodily function such as oxygenation, food absorption, detoxification and the generation of nerve impulses all happen at the cell wall by the movement of positive and negative particles across it. Each cell depends on life-supporting supplies, including oxygen, water, glucose and protein. Waste products such as carbon dioxide and urine require disposal. Like a huge metropolis the body continues growing, replicating, defending and repairing itself. It does this whether we are in a coma, sleeping, dreaming or awake.

Consider the ingenuity of the immune system. T-cells move through the body scanning for and eliminating dangerous material. They contain the knowledge of what is 'me' and what is 'not me', then act accordingly. We're not awakened in the middle of the night by the chief T-cell seeking an executive decision as to whether or not to destroy the alien. In the same way everything from the regulation of our heartbeat, to the repair of our cells in the event of damage is guided by an organising power outside my intellectual control.

What do you think would happen if you were left in charge of your heartbeat and the phone rang — a fatal distraction? It is just as well that we are not conscious of the intelligence watching over us. It is a power outside our awareness — the life-force that is expressed in us as our personalised spark of life. Our physical life literally starts with the life-force entering us and ends with it leaving us.

The obvious question is that if we are so well looked after by the life-force, how come Mary's, John's and Julian's mental lives are no longer 'on-line'? Why are their mental lives not supported by this intelligence as is their immune system? Obviously balance has been lost and their expression of the life-force, at least at some levels, has become skewed. So what has caused this shift? Why is it expressing itself in different ways in each of them? What is behind it all? Could there be more here than meets the eye?

LET'S ASK OUR PANEL OF EXPERTS

The understanding of how the mind works, like the various reflections on the nature of life and spirit, has occupied the greatest minds for thousands of years and will no doubt continue to do so. Psychological distress, because it involves the mind, is like spirit in that it is abstract in nature. As such it is more difficult to pin down by the experts than are other medical problems, such as a dysfunctional heart or diabetes.

We have created a fictitious panel of experts, to help us to introduce some of the views currently held by healers working in different ways with the psychologically distressed. Some of their interpretations and insights are not usually found together in one book and are generally excluded from the world of psychiatry.

We have included on the panel only some of the healers whose fields of expertise we have collaborated with in our

clinical practice through the years and whose assistance we
have found invaluable. We respectfully honour the work of
those in disciplines which we have not included or with whom
we have not yet had the opportunity to join forces. We favour
the mind-body-spirit approach and consequently have chosen
to give a greater voice to panel members of that persuasion.

The panel will include a psychiatrist, a psychologist, an energy therapist, a homeopath, a spiritual healer and a specialist in the
field of mind-brain chemistry. During our training in hospital
medicine, consultations were frequently held around the bedside
between a number of experts whose opinion was sought relative
to treatment. In a similar way we will ask our panel to 'take a
look' at a number of individuals 'as if' they were real patients, to
give you a feel for the variety of ways of viewing the same psychiatric problem. They will appear as needed throughout the
book. We have included Joe, from the sandwich bar, in our panel
to represent local knowledge of some of the characters and the
likely commonplace interpretations of their behaviours.

The Panel's View of Mary's Panic Attack

Joe (layperson): has been working in his sandwich bar for years
and regards himself as an 'expert' on human relationships.
One thing he knows is that lately Mary has been acting differ-
ently. Some days she has been impatient, snappy and pushy and
on others distant and self-absorbed. If he didn't know her so
well, he would swear it was a totally different girl he was seeing these days.

Ruth (psychotherapist): looking at Mary's recent irritable
and edgy behaviour, thinks 'She is obviously panicky and trying
her best to cover it up. What she needs to do is get in touch
with her feelings of inadequacy, track back and look at where
they started in childhood and learn to substitute her negative
mindset with a more empowering one — challenging her pho-
bic behaviours instead of giving in to them.'

Dr Henry (psychiatrist): has formed the opinion that Mary
suffers from panic disorder. In his book it is a chemical imbalance which, he predicts, will lead to severe agoraphobia and
depression if not treated with medication. Unlike Ruth, who
locates Mary's problem in her values, attitudes and beliefs — i.e.
her mind or 'software' — Henry sees it as a disease in her brain
or 'hardware'.

Jackie (energy therapist): has been formulating her own interpretation of what is 'wrong' with Mary. She can see, through higher sense perception, Mary's aura which is formed from the electromagnetic field around her body and her seven chakras. (see Appendix.) Jackie notices the changes in Mary's energy as she approaches the top of the queue. This reflects the overall state of imbalance or interference in the organisation of her field. It is obvious to her that Mary's levels of fear are rising and reaching panic proportions. Jackie's opinion is 'If she doesn't get out of here soon she's going to have a panic attack. Her feeling of not being safe or secure is coming from a third chakra issue, her centre of personal power in her solar plexus. The butterflies and the knot in her stomach are evidence of this.'

Patrick (spiritual healer): takes a 'big picture' reading of the whole thing. For years now he has been having clairvoyant psychic experiences. It makes perfect sense to him that the scientists and the mystics are coming up with the same answer; that there is a universal consciousness or divine intention which brought everything into existence.

Through his ability to receive information from other realms of consciousness Patrick understands how energy created matter and how matter, through a series of integrating twists and turns — amino acid by amino acid, cell by cell — became life. From this perspective he sees Mary as a spiritual being having a human experience, her soul having become embodied with an agenda or plan which will unfold over the course of her lifetime.

He sees her soul journey as a process of learning new ways of reacting to situations and in so doing changing her karmic patterns. He understands these to be her reactions, her layers of conditioned responses, whether mental, emotional or behavioural, to a whole variety of experiences she has faced in her past — either in this lifetime or a previous one. He believes that Mary is now being presented with an opportunity to learn through her panic attacks, to overcome her fears by becoming more conscious of their source. Only by witnessing such disempowering beliefs can she change and master them.

Patrick sees the soul journey as a continuous process of reincarnation in different human forms. Constantly evolving, through the gathering of knowledge and information gained through experience — not unlike the DNA story. He believes that, when our material part dies the knowledge gained returns to the soul pool, to be used again by other entities. Through the cycle of birth, death and rebirth known as reincarnation, the human being evolves toward God-consciousness or union with the cosmic mind. He is reminded of Teilhard de Chardin, the great philosopher who saw the human being as being irresistibly drawn to form one single whole, the 'noosphere'.

He can see the different levels involved in Mary's make-up, her entire multidimensional anatomy. How her soul is reflected in every wave, molecule and cell of her body. He is aware of her chakras and electromagnetic energy field, the fearful thoughts and images she is running, the adrenaline cascade, her racing heart, her sweaty palms and the shallow breathing. He knows, like Jackie, that a full-blown panic attack is imminent, a symptom of her disquiet. He thinks, 'Small wonder that psychiatry has its roots in the words *psyche* meaning "soul" and *iatriea* meaning "healing". Yet where is she going to find such a "soul healer" who can place her on her soul's time line and see what issues from past lives are contributing to her deep sense of insecurity, of which her panic is the mere tip of the iceberg?'

We can see from our panel of experts that their views of Mary vary and are a reflection of their own database. As the philosopher Wittgenstein said, 'When all you have is a hammer, everything looks like a nail.' Let's assemble our panel and ask them to bring their toolboxes and take a look at John and Julian.

The Panel's View of John's Schizophrenic State

They find John in his bedroom, sleeping off another night of oneness experiences. In such moments he inhabits a state of consciousness in which he loses all sense of connection with the thoughts and feelings by which he traditionally knows himself. That 'old' John, has been replaced by a newer experience, born within his psychotic state. He now has an inner knowing that he is part of the universal cosmic mind, which he understands to be 'that which is behind everything'. Occasionally he laughs aloud at the enormity of that comprehension.

When pressed for an explanation by his mother as to what he is laughing at he replies, 'We're all in the flow of the lifeforce, so we've nothing to worry about. Fighting it is like trying to stop a tidal wave with your hand.' He cannot understand why his family can't grasp what his experiences mean. He knows they don't because they keep pestering him about work and his eccentric behaviours. His six-year-old sister has told him that he is 'mad' and his father has threatened to call the doctor and have him committed to the local psychiatric hospital.

Joe (layperson): reflects that John was always a shy, sensitive boy, who lived in the shadow of his older brother Peter, who was John's minder. 'He'd come in looking for a sandwich and was never able to look you in the eye. Oversensitive by far.'

Ruth (psychotherapist): is aware that he was bullied around the neighbourhood and called names. 'After his brother Peter got killed on the motorbike he didn't stand a chance. He had nobody to protect him and his father was never at home. As a way of coping he became even more isolated, feeling safer and more secure in his own company. He found school too demanding and felt so anxious there he could never really learn anything much. If he'd been identified earlier as being at risk, he might have done well. But then extreme shyness isn't on the 'at risk' list in the same way that dyslexia is. More's the pity.'

Dr Henry (psychiatrist): has the view that John is suffering from schizophrenia and at this stage he requires immediate hospitalisation. 'He needs anti-psychotic medication to dampen down his florid symptoms. He'll probably be on some sort of medication for the rest of his life and will always need a sheltered environment.'

Jackie (energy therapist): gives her opinion. 'From what I see all his energy has moved up to his seventh or crown chakra, his spiritual one. It's as if he's spinning in outer space, he's so out of his body. That's because, without actually knowing it, he's been moving energy away from his lower chakras for years. They're the ones that give us the skills to deal with everyday life at a raw survival level. He's never built up any confidence in that area. That's why he has difficulty feeling secure. All his life he's been afraid and it's not the kind of fear that a child can explain to adults.

'He's oversensitive, has always felt misunderstood and has never gelled with his peers. His aura is so porous that everything affects him deeply. No wonder he had to hide behind his brother Peter. Kids like John just can't take the knocks on the earth plane and spend all of their time trying to get back to the cosmic realm where they feel safe. He's just been like a lost soul.'

Patrick (spiritual healer): also coming from the energetic perspective feels that 'While medication can stop him spinning and bring him back into this reality, if he's not made to feel safe, regardless of whatever medication he's on, he'll only go out again. In an ideal world he would spend a long time in the safety of a therapeutic community, among people of his own age, with specialised therapists on hand. With such a buffer between himself and the outside world, he might begin to feel safe and learn how to keep his energy grounded.

'Looking at the span of his past lifetimes,' continues Patrick, 'it's my understanding that he has had many experiences that have made him fearful of the earth plane. In this incarnation his karmic task is to learn ways to be at home here, to remain more present. His symptoms are an expression of his soul pain as he tries to do that. His dilemma is whether to stay or not to stay. For John, putting down roots is not an easy task and difficult for him to do alone. This psychotic break is what I would call a spiritual emergency.'

The Panel's View of Julian's Manic Episode

Backstage at Julian's concert Joe (layperson) makes the following observation: 'This is his big night. It's now or never. He's been practising morning, noon and night. Hasn't been seen for weeks. As a child he was always so confident. He'd be in my place with his mother and she'd be crowing about his next concert and how he was going to take the place by storm. 'He's such a genius,' she'd say, 'everyone says he has a brilliant future. He'll make us all so proud.'

As Julian walks off the stage in a triumphal state, he makes the flamboyant announcement, 'You are looking at the greatest pianist of all time — the Archangel Gabriel in person.' Looking at him, **Dr Henry (psychiatrist)** makes his diagnosis. 'He's gone psychotic! He's experiencing a manic break. The only thing that'll stop it is hospitalisation and high doses of medication.'

Ruth (psychotherapist): has this interpretation of why he has become elated. 'He's overcompensated for his fear of failure by trying too hard. He's been winding himself up in his determination to be a success, burning the candle at both ends, with a tunnel-vision attitude toward his goal. No way was he going to fail this time!'

Jackie (energy therapist): relates what she saw while he was on stage. 'His aura was huge coming up to the crescendo. Most of his energy was concentrated in his sixth chakra. No wonder he plugged into the Archangel Gabriel, that's where the powerful archetypes are experienced. Some manics take on the persona of famous or powerful people, such as Buddha or Jesus, depending on their belief system. Gabriel was an excellent choice as it suited Messiaen's 'The Ascension' piece very well!

'Energetically he turned his fear of failure into success by shifting his energy upwards. Since he was small he was primed with all that 'genius' stuff and his obvious talent got blown out of all proportion. It's so ironic, setbacks were not part of his repertoire. It's easier to be a big fish in a small pond, but Paris was shark-infested waters. It was the first time Julian experienced not being top dog and he couldn't handle it. You could say he cooked the books! This happened through the concentration of energy in his sixth chakra, his third eye, where in a way you can make your dreams come true. That's why when he looks at himself through it, everything gets magnified, he becomes larger than life, the greatest success ever.'

Patrick (spiritual healer): says 'His karmic task this life-time is to learn to be ordinary, to handle failure and to accept imperfection. For many incarnations he was obsessed with success at any cost and held positions of real power. His word was law. Many times he left a trail of destruction behind him. This manic episode will also cause a lot of collateral damage, although on a smaller scale. It will finally force him to realise that you can pay too high a price for success. In this way his consciousness will expand and he will be able to stand back and become more of a witness to his life. This is the position from which free will and conscious choices come more easily and from which connection to our spiritual journey is established.

'If the witness is not developed, if we remain unaware, if we don't learn to observe ourselves, how can we change our behaviours? We can't change something until we know it exists. Spiritual growth depends on this awareness. Julian currently has no insight into his situation. He is merely being swept away by the power of his own energy. He refuses to see reality as it is, only as he'd like it to be. His greatest spiritual learning will happen when this manic episode inevitably burns out and he becomes aware of the chaos he has created. Through this experience his witness will be born.'

Having listened to our panel of experts we can see that each one has their own specific 'window on the world'. Their interpretations are a reflection of their experience and training. Within the larger scheme of things all are valid.

SECTION 2

CHAPTER 5 — SCHIZOPHRENIA

Keynote: Lost in Space

S chizophrenia — **what a word!** When asked what it means, we trot out expressions like split personality, crazy, mad, insane, loony, nutcase, a screw loose, round the bend, not the full deck, off the wall, etc. The images that float in, the movies that our minds begin to run, build a picture of a person who laughs to themselves, has conversations with people who aren't there, sits rocking in a corner, makes strange gesticulations, walks in an odd way, seems oblivious to others, looks like a down-and-out and does bizarre things like standing in the middle of the road directing traffic.

One thing is certain, if we met this person on the street we wouldn't want to engage them and we would dread becoming like them. We certainly wouldn't want to bring them home. Like a country that nobody wants to visit, schizophrenia has a public face that scares us away — it has bad press. Our images of a schizophrenic are quick snapshot views. Like a tourist on a bus, we have taken photos of the natives without ever getting out and actually talking to one. But where do these snapshots come from, given that very few of us have actually met a schizophrenic? They have to have come from somewhere: stereotypical caricatures acted out in movies, TV, theatre, novels etc. Given that a snapshot is only an impression, a surface view, how much can it really tell us about what is going on behind the scenes?

Let's return to John and pick it up from where the experts left off. Already we have a fair idea of the ingredients that have created the present-day John. He is a real human being who has found himself at the far end of the sanity-insanity spectrum and he is typical of one who has recently entered the schizophrenic state — i.e. on the surface.

Walk into any Irish country pub as a tourist and you will get a typical impression of Irish drinkers, in other words, your snapshot view. You know absolutely nothing about the millions of variables that have gone into the composition of each individual drinker. Their background is a blank. If you were to get to know each one individually, you would know that they are more dissimilar from each other than similar. The same is true

of your so-called 'typical' schizophrenic. Having said that, schizophrenics have in common many shared characteristics, just like
the drinkers.

Before we paint the picture it seems appropriate to define
our subject. First the classical dictionary definition:

Schizophrenia *is a psychotic mental disorder characterised
by a breakdown in the relation between thoughts, feelings and
actions, usually accompanied by withdrawal from social activity and the occurrence of delusions and hallucinations.*

(The origin of this term comes from the Greek *skhizein*
meaning 'to split or divide' and from the old English 'to shed',
'to separate' or 'to cast off' and from the Greek *phren* meaning
'mind'.)

Since this definition contains the words psychotic, delusions
and hallucinations, further clarification is required.

Psychosis *is a severe mental illness or derangement or disorder involving a loss of contact with reality frequently with hallucinations or delusions, or altered thought processes.*

Hallucination *is the apparent perception of an external
object or sensory input when no such object or stimulus is present (seeing things, hearing voices).*

Delusion *is a false impression or opinion not shared by
others.*

Let us translate these classical definitions into a form which
is less intimidating and is more descriptive of the 'inner voice'
or experience of schizophrenics themselves. For example, John
has left earthbound existence, leaving his mind-body behind
and is in spirit form travelling around the cosmos having a 'oneness' experience. (He is 'out of his mind'.) John is now psychotic. He has separated from, cast off, split and divided from
his old reality; the one that his parents, the rest of us and ultimately his psychiatrist inhabit. Naturally his thought processes
are altered. He is like an astronaut on Saturn trying to convey
what he is experiencing; it is a case of 'you had to be there'. Of
course John is seeing things, hearing things and is unable to
share them with others.

The nearest most of us will ever come to experiencing
where John is, is when we dream. We see things, hear voices,
smell, touch and taste. We have sex with people we have never
met before and can even have better orgasms than we do in
this reality. Within the world of the classical definitions we are
actively psychotic. Our partner in bed beside us hasn't a clue
what we are talking about, who we are talking to, what our

twistings and turnings are about and cannot see the lover in our arms. Their visual absence to our partner doesn't invalidate their existence to us. Without being oversimplistic, we can come out of our psychotic dream state when the alarm rings and end it. However, John experiences his dreams in waking consciousness. In other words he is caught up in a continuous daydream.

A PORTRAIT OF A TYPICAL SCHIZOPHRENIC

Contrary to popular opinion, the onset of schizophrenia is not sudden. It is not the case that one day everything is normal and the next day one is experiencing a schizophrenic state. The condition develops slowly over time; it is an integral part and an expression of the person's life history. It is a process rather than a sudden event.

Schizophrenia is more understandable if seen as having two phases.

1. The Pre-psychotic Phase

- Timidity, fragility, hypersensitivity and being on the edge of group activities are features found in early childhood.
- During the teenage years schizophrenics behave as if they do not want to be here, as if too sensitive for this world. Engagement in eccentric loner behaviours and interests is safer than the rough and tumble of team sports. The social identity achieved through group activities that adolescents engage in such as music, socialising, experimenting with recreational substances, making shapes at the opposite sex, fitting in with a group 'look' and testing limits, is beyond their range of skills and puts them outside their comfort zone.
- This lack of fit with their peers is often unsympathetically fed back to them through indifference, ridicule, bullying and name-calling. They can find themselves jeered at, with innuendoes made about their sexual orientation. As the teenage years go by, they find themselves more and more marginalised, alienated and left out of things, which only serves to reinforce their sense of difference.

- **Poor performance at school** is commonplace because of distractibility, daydreaming and finding school content unengaging.
- **Particularly from early adolescent life**, parents, siblings, relatives and family friends note an idiosyncratic and aloof style of behaviour. Their conversational content can be strikingly different and hard to connect with. They are often described as 'odd'.
- **Educational and social milestones** can be out of their reach, once again reflecting their poor social skills. Graduation from school, entering college, forming a romantic relationship, maintaining a social life with peers and achieving independence from parents is fraught with difficulty.
- **Time-wise they fall behind the group**, which becomes more noticeable as early adult life commences. A failed rite of passage is now evident both to themselves and those around them. Serious questions and worries now start to arise in the minds of their parents.
- **As their fear intensifies** their nervous behaviour increases and they can have angry outbursts when their social avoidance strategies are challenged. Consequently they create a climate where — for the sake of peace — their eccentric routines are begrudgingly tolerated. Paradoxically now more powerful, they are allowed drop out of school, college and like John, jobs. Frequently parents throw their eyes up to heaven and retreat in confusion.
- **Adrift from the routine of a social role**, they disconnect from prior personal routines and habits. They often sleep during the day and are up at night, eat on their own and neglect personal hygiene and appearance. At this stage it's not uncommon for them to form relationships with other social drifters, go missing, sleep rough and become less and less accountable for their behaviours.

2. The Psychotic Phase

- **This phase unquestionably begins** when the workings of the inner world finally take over. Fantasy has become reality and the waking dream, with its exquisitely unique chemistry, bombards the schizophrenic with stimuli from within. The analogy that comes closest to this state is that of a sleepwalker on a grand scale. Their internal images, how they experience them and their complementary or matching behaviours, close sufferers off from the outside world, just like the sleepwalker. Unlike the sleepwalker, however, who snaps out of it when disturbed by an outsider, our psychotic does not. The walking-waking-dream state continues to run and run. The outside 'intruder' is experienced and interpreted according to their internal universe.

- **A mismatch occurs** between the sufferer's internal universe and the external reality. When forced to interface with others, schizophrenics can become frightened, paranoid (see Chapter 11 — Paranoia), irritable and can aggressively assert their wish to be left undisturbed. Any appeals to think, act, or feel to the contrary are ignored. Their behaviours understandably fit with their own belief system and empathy with others gets lost. As time progresses, so unique, idiosyncratic and exclusive does the schizophrenic's world become that there is very little common ground left. Hallucinations (from the Latin *allucinari* meaning 'to wander in one's mind') reinforces and validates their alienation as well as strengthening the division between them and the outside world. (In energy terms the sixth chakra holds our interpretative filtering system imbued with the symbols, beliefs and values of our culture. Any energetic information processed by it will be skewed and coloured by this bias. For example, a schizophrenic raised in the Christian tradition is unlikely to translate their energetic input from the seventh chakra into forms and archetypes which belong to the spiritual traditions of the North American Indian, the Australian Aborigine or the Hindu. In other words, *the expression of the energy sensed at the seventh chakra is interpreted through the eyes and ears of the sixth chakra, which is a reflection of their culture.*)

- **Verbal communication is as awkward** as it might be between a Martian and an earthling. The content is often jumbled, disordered, nonsensical, out-of-context and repetitious. The term 'word salad' best describes this phenomenon. Accompanying this there can be 'pressure of speech' which reflects the extent of their bombardment internally by a flood of disorganised information.

- **It is at this point** that schizophrenia is professionally diagnosed. But as we can see, it has been a long time coming.

St Jude's Observation Ward

John is sleeping off heavy doses of anti-psychotic medication on day three of his admission.

Let's Ask Our Panel of Experts

Joe (layperson): 'He's finally in the right place, this last week has been hell for the whole family. He was like the character in the movie *Birdy*, perched on the end of his bed staring out of the window into space, laughing and gibbering to himself. His poor mother was demented trying to get him to come out of his bedroom and eat something. His younger sister was afraid to bring her friends into the house in case he'd embarrass her. As for his father, he was relieved that finally action had been taken and John was going to get treatment.'

Ruth (psychotherapist): 'It's always difficult for a family to acknowledge that one of its members has crossed the line into madness. Many live with eccentric and disruptive behaviours for years hoping that they will 'grow out of it' or that it will 'go away'. He's going to need an awful lot of aftercare. He's never had a solid sense of himself — a poor ego. Leaky boundaries, no wonder he could never feel safe. After Peter was killed he felt even more exposed and vulnerable and lived in fear of being invaded by the energy of others. His best coping strategy was to hide himself away and make a world of his own. In the end it just took him over.'

Dr Henry (psychiatrist): 'The mainstream medical view is that it is an underlying organic disease within John's brain which is creating his schizophrenic state. We believe that one day the gene responsible for schizophrenia will be discovered.'

Jackie (energy therapist): 'Like I was saying when we all gathered in his bedroom, I could see then that he was going to lift completely out of his body and go into orbit. Wasn't all his energy concentrated in his seventh chakra? (See Appendix.) The energetic story of schizophrenia, of which John is a good example, primarily relates to the first, sixth and seventh chakras.

'The first chakra is formed in the intrauterine phase and the first twelve months of life. The infant's first energetic task is to firmly implant in the physical world, in other words make a commitment to be here. This forms the bedrock upon which the child builds the rest of its life. In energy language we call this 'being grounded'. Without this foundation the child does not have a sense of feeling stable, safe or secure. If this healthy energetic 'skin' or 'boundary' is not in place, essential self-definition does not occur. This means that in the process of growing up the child can feel overwhelmed, invaded and threatened by the stronger energies of others.

'Fearing this, they retreat as it were to 'higher ground', withdrawing their energy to the upper chakras, creating a mind-body split which is the fundamental underpinning of the pre-psychotic phase. In doing this, the lower chakras — i.e. the first, second and third — which are those responsible for physical, emotional and ego identity, don't mature properly. When these vital milestones are omitted, kids like this have little interest in bodily activities or in participating as individuals. Just like John they show little enthusiasm for physical activities, sexual exploration or group pursuits. It's easy to see how their eccentricities and loner behaviours predominate as their interests and their energies lie in the non-physical and they live more in their heads. This marked difference marks them as outsiders and leaves them wide open to ridicule.

'One of the biggest problems for John was that his seventh chakra was functioning like a portal through which he was accessing oneness and unity. If he was a Tibetan monk, he would have achieved the goal of his life — boundlessness. That's what all the great mystics were seeking. The only difference between them and John was that they had firmly installed the wisdom chips and other vital pieces of software to interpret that extraordinary experience and integrate it into their lives. In other words their sixth chakra (the centre of understanding) was actively seeking the oneness experience and was therefore ready for it — enabled by years of teaching, prayer and meditation. Same experience — different result. They were trained to handle unity consciousness — unsolvable Zen koans (problems with no logical solutions) like 'What's the sound of one hand clapping?' — which paved the way for the nature of the 'oneness' experience which is almost impossible to verbalise.

'There's one extra piece to this. When John's sixth chakra started to download the experiences of his seventh, he filtered it through his ordinary, socially constructed mindset in keeping with the conditioning of his culture. The experience was just too big to integrate. It was like lightning hitting a house and, having no way of grounding, it blew his mind. When he tried to put words on it, it came out all gobbledygook.'

Professor Moore (mind-brain specialist): 'My expertise is in the area of mind-brain chemistry. In my field, vibrational medicine, we study the behaviour of electromagnetic waves and their particle equivalent in the form of chemical molecules. We know from quantum physics that wave and particle are interchangeable, thoughts create chemistry and vice versa. The best way of understanding a thought is as an impulse of energy and information, which can change matter in the same way that the remote control can change the stations on a TV set.

'Thoughts are very powerful, they literally create the way we are — they create our world. Everything that has ever been created by human beings has first existed at the level of thought — everything. From the first fire to the latest space station — we are what we think. The body itself doesn't decide on the state it'll be in any more than the TV picks its own stations. As I was saying, our thoughts act like buttons on the remote. They are causal and the experiences they create are the effects. If you think peaceful thoughts you'll have the 'peace channel' being experienced in the body. Happy thoughts make happy molecules. If your thoughts are fearful you'll have the 'panic channel'. Thoughts which are predominantly, 'I don't want to be here', can dictate that the 'psychotic channel' is the one you're experiencing.

'John has been pressing that button for most of his life and has created the clinical state of schizophrenia. While medication will dampen down John's florid symptoms it will not cure him because the origin of his problem is at the level of his ideas — his software. It is so important to understand that psychoactive medication can at best, only attempt to deal with the effects. There is nothing wrong with John's brain — his hardware. Insisting that this is the case is like calling the TV repair man when you don't like the programmes showing.

'The chemistry produced during schizophrenic experiences and transcendental states have much in common. The development of quantum physics is such that we have now reached the point where the scientists and the mystics can agree as to the nature of reality. It makes sense to me that we are spiritual beings having human experiences.'

Patrick (spiritual healer): 'John's mind-brain chemistry has similarities with the transcendental states produced by the ingestion of hallucinogenic plants in ancient civilisations. For thousands of years the Indians in the upper Amazon have been using them, referring to them as 'plants of the gods'. These naturally occurring hallucinogenic substances can alter the consciousness of the mind, giving the user an experience of the divine. In our western medical framework the same state is called schizophrenia. In the case of the Indians the chemical is consciously ingested, while in the case of schizophrenics like John it is naturally but unconsciously created.

'Also naturally created, but in a conscious way, is the chemistry associated with the rare transcendental moments during meditation known as 'enlightenment', 'bliss' and 'God consciousness'. What the native Indians and the meditators have in common is that these activities are culturally embraced, actively fostered and taught. As such, the content of their oneness experiences can be placed within an understandable framework by the elders, the shaman and the spiritual teacher. In Old Irish culture, people who went mad were called 'duine le dia' — people with God — which implied that there was an understanding that their experiences were transcendental in nature and were respected. This holds true in certain parts of present-day India.

'Contrast this with John who somehow, accidentally through his need to feel safe, has shifted his energy upwards and as a result altered his chemical profile. This gave him a way of leaving everyday reality and moving 'with the gods'. What makes him different from the Indians and the meditators is that he did not seek such a state, was unprepared for it, cannot voluntarily turn it off and only has a pathological medical framework within which to interpret it. It's not as simple as waiting for the effect of the plant to wear off, or the sound of a gong to distract him.

'Think about it. If John, or others like him, actually found the altered state of consciousness frightening, they might be terrified by it and worse, feel that they might not be able to end it — enter paranoia. (See Chapter 11 — Paranoia.) Experiences of this magnitude, like any other, can be interpreted as good or bad. Ultimately the experience you have would reflect your value system.

'Wouldn't the shaman or abbot who found John wandering in the jungle or the cloister make a completely different interpretation of his experience than his white-coated Harvardschooled psychiatrist? This is where I would disagree with psychiatrists who do not value the vital role of psychotherapy. After John's psychosis is contained and dampened down with medication, he will need an opportunity to make sense of what's happened to him — to understand it.

'When a human being has been through an unusual or traumatic experience such as space travel, hostage situations, kidnapping, rape, war, train and plane crashes, earthquakes, etc. debriefing should be the norm. Increasingly this is the case. This allows the individual to put words on their experiences and the accompanying images and feelings. Sharing these and having them understood helps to put a framework on them. Downloading the unspeakable into words helps to put a concrete form on it, which can be 'filed' or integrated into the prior self. Many of these debriefings take place in controlled environments over days and sometimes weeks.

'To those who have returned from a schizophrenic state, they feel that the experience they've had is extraordinary. They have travelled beyond the traditional boundaries of finite consciousness into the boundlessness of infinity. They were alone having the experience. The content was unique and happened in a different time zone, but remains as 'real' as the fingers on their hands. Having the content of that reality ignored and written off as if it never happened, compounds their bewilderment.

'In general, every detail of the psychotic experience is remembered. A perfect memory trace is laid down. They need to be helped to express this in language, art, drama or some other form so that it gets released. If this doesn't happen the experience isn't integrated. It sits in the mind as a piece of alien software, waiting to be loaded and run again and again. Just like a flashback only more intense and prolonged.

'Long term use of medication freezes the experience, introduces side effects and in addition saps the energy that would otherwise be available for the difficult task of rebuilding their lives. If the medication is stopped, the experience seeps out and recurs, seducing them back to the altered state, especially if it was a pleasant one. In psychiatric terminology this is called a 'relapse'. I see it as a 'release' and a re-connection to the boundless. Once again, as they come out of the psychosis an opportunity for debriefing presents itself. This usually doesn't happen and the lifelong use of medication becomes inevitable. In this way they're maintained at a threshold below the experience, not psychotic but not cured either — frozen between the worlds and trapped in the twilight zone. From the soul's perspective, what greater tragedy could occur than to live this lifetime under the cloud of a hazy, chemically-induced, medicated state? This creates even further distance from his soul journey. The expert's stance 'we don't want to talk about it' locks the individual permanently into this state — they can't move on. Years later, the more time they spend in this limbo the less possibility there is of them ever integrating into reality.

'Demystification of his boundless experience is necessary for John. That it had an understandable logic, a clear background and a lead-up that can explain why it happened at all. More importantly, this knowledge can give him choices and a sense of control regarding the future. Recognising the patterns and ingredients that were in play prior to his psychotic break would make John an active agent, a player in his own healing. In terms of changing karmic patterns, he would now be able to use that quintessentially human quality — free will.

'When I look at the soul journey of the Johns of this world, what I see is that the initial point of difficulty starts with the process of incarnation — the point where the soul or spirit enters the physical body. For a multitude of karmic reasons their spirit is unwilling to fully commit to the journey on the physical plane and maintains a longing to return to its source. In this way they always maintain a foot in both worlds with split intention — whether to stay or to go. Since they can't leave physically unless they commit suicide, they move their energy upwards, concentrating it as we have said in the top chakras and in so doing avoid being fully 'here'.

'If, as I have said, John's karmic task is to commit to this reality through the use of his free will, then it's ironic that the medicated state on which he is maintained, freezes it. In terms of learning, going through the psychotic experience will have been for nothing if he's offered no opportunity for transformation. This is what psychotherapy or soul healing is all about.'

Dr Clarke (homeopath): 'It's for this very reason that homeopathy has its place. If a shy introverted boy like John had been identified earlier according to his constitutional nature or state, it may have reduced his levels of fear enough to make it more comfortable for him to be here. Homeopathic remedies work vibrationally at all levels of the energy field — in other words the mind-body-spirit dimensions.

'If a psychotherapeutic programme is ever created for John, remedies can help to bring his life-force back into a state of balance by changing its frequency. Anti-psychotic medication as used in psychiatric practice are crucial in the short term as it terminates the psychotic episode. It does this by shutting down the excessive energy at the sixth and seventh chakras. In the long term, however, it can be counter-productive as it paralyses consciousness and as Patrick has said, free will.

'It is only a question of time before the disciplines which have an energetic basis, such as psychotherapy, bodywork, acupuncture, energy work and homeopathy, will integrate to create a holistic approach to psychological distress. It is my vision that healing centres with this ethos will emerge.

'A new paradigm in psychiatry is long overdue. It's obvious that the current system isn't working. Let's be honest, if psychoactive medication cured rather than contained the problem, psychiatric outpatient departments and hospitals would be empty. Getting the news that you have a disorder that is beyond your control, chemical in origin, possibly lifelong and one that requires daily medication to keep it at bay is in my view a serious obstruction to healing because it's so disempowering. People give up if there's no hope. For many this is the beginning of life as a chemical cripple.

'The argument that schizophrenia is genetically transmitted is not only depressing but highly questionable. It's common sense to me that since schizophrenics don't tend to engage in intimate relationships or have children, the so-called genetic pool should have long become extinct. Relying on this theory as a cause diverts valuable research money from holistic approaches.'

CHAPTER 6 — MANIA

Keynote: A Flight into Grandeur

Mania and schizophrenia are often confused because they both conjure up images of madness. In fact they have almost nothing in common except the umbrella term 'psychosis', meaning *an altered state of consciousness*. They are as different as chalk and cheese, night and day.

So, what is the difference? They are different in terms of cause, personality type, speed and manner of onset, thought content and behaviour, chemical and energetic profile, their clinical course and outcome.

At its very core, mania is an unconscious defence against failure. Feeling ordinary, vulnerable and out of control are not part of the mania mindset. Mania-sufferers like to be extraordinary, invulnerable and on top. They reject the 'down' position and will distort any evidence that it is on the horizon — overcompensating in the opposite direction. Their last-ditch efforts to 'pull it off' in the face of all objective evidence to the contrary, are legendary. This behaviour is akin to rearranging the deckchairs on the sinking *Titanic*, encouraging the dance-band to play their hearts out while they keep the champagne flowing!

Once mania is seen as a manoeuvre to essentially avoid, deny and escape from the feelings of setback, disappointment and failure which are so much a part of everyday life for all of us; then the behaviours it provokes begins to make sense.

The schizophrenic by contrast is shy, hypersensitive, socially awkward and, as mentioned in the chapter on schizophrenia, noticeably different from his or her siblings and peers. Schizophrenics prefer solitary pursuits, they stay on the edge of the group, they are introverted and generally do not fit in. Onset of the condition is so slow and insidious that it is only in retrospect that family members recognise there may have been a problem of a longstanding nature.

A PORTRAIT OF MANIA

The Predicament on the Horizon

In contrast to the young schizophrenic, the pre-manic years are relatively trouble free. No shrinking violets, mania-sufferers are more often high achievers, socially skilled, confident, pro-active, competitive and familiar with success. They are good all-rounders and some may well be voted in their class as being the 'most likely to succeed'. They enter the world of work full of promise because of this apparent head start. Naïvety and wishful-thinking can compound the problem in some. The first sign of a psychological hiccup can come therefore as a total shock to patient and family alike. Their game plan for the future was one of continued success! To return to the analogy of the *Titanic*, their predicted life seemed unsinkable and Plan B, the need for lifeboats, was never considered.

How they look to others is important to them: the public gaze, material things, getting ahead and the need for power and approval is crucial to their identity (externally referred). They are often larger than life, the life and soul of the party and are well liked. Their bonhomie and extrovert nature attracts people to them. When it comes to having their own needs met, they expect doors to be opened for them and see no reason why they should not be facilitated.

They expect others to give their all and share enthusiastically in their dreams and visions. If challenged on practicalities they become annoyed, impatient and frustrated. Familiar with the high-horse position, if obstructed they can ride rough-shod over colleagues, family and friends. A setback is not on their agenda. They are survivors at all costs.

When a setback occurs, the predicament it throws up will illicit an exaggerated response in this pre-manic group. While others may sympathise with them, few appreciate the depth and intensity of their newly felt vulnerable feelings as their ego is unquestionably challenged for the first time. Typical setbacks might include not achieving the expected result in an exam, missing a promotion, a broken romance and in general losing face and not pulling it off. What would be experienced as a minor obstacle to others becomes an earthquake to them in psychological terms. It is as though they have put everything, even their very personhood, on the line. The reverberations are huge and prove too much for their systems to handle.

Rather than experience feelings of failure, the incoming evidence is rejected and distorted by the mania mindset and the blame for setbacks is projected onto others. They contrive explanations which free them from any personal responsibility — in other words they *cook the books*. Reasons and rationalisations are dragged up to offload responsibility for the failure.

This has the unfortunate consequence that the core problem is never addressed and the slide downwards continues. A point is inevitably reached where denial can no longer hide the reality of the situation and they are forced to acknowledge that a failure is imminent. When the dam bursts and the truth of the situation is no longer avoidable, the personal lie starts to break down.

There are recognisable phases to the manic process akin to the launching of a rocket into space, its orbiting and its return, re-entry, crash landing and fallout.

Max, a successful, high profile rally driver was invited into a partnership with an older man who specialised in retailing classic cars. The company was extremely successful and his family enjoyed a lavish lifestyle. Following the partner's death, Max, who had never managed the financial side of the business, started to make serious financial errors of judgement. Ultimately, with the banks foreclosing, he refused to heed the advice of friends and family that unless he restructured the business by selling off non-profit-making outlets he would be soon be bankrupt. This he could not accept and avidly sought new investors, becoming even more flamboyant in his lifestyle. After six months of extravagant overspending and failing to see the writing on the wall, the company was forced into bankruptcy and he was treated for his first manic episode.

THE LAUNCH PAD

Staring failure in the face, mania-sufferers move rapidly in the opposite direction, back to the success end of the success-failure spectrum. In this way they impress upon themselves, as well as trying to impress upon others, that they are still in control — proving this by overcompensating.

There is a noticeable speeding up of thoughts and behaviours. Subjectively they feel a surge of energy, power and invincibility. It is as if they have become the Greek character Sisyphus, who has suddenly found the extra strength to push the boulder over the ridge of the mountain and down the other side, finally freeing himself from repeated failures. There is an air of triumphalism — anything is possible!

This is the stage where the psychotic break has not yet occurred, but is imminent. It is an exaggerated and magnified version of themselves on top form — a caricature. As they move closer to the launch pad, the possibility of aborting the mission rapidly fades.

Launch Pad Symptoms

- **Unstoppable rapid-fire speech**, full of inflated high sounding rhetoric. They are incapable of listening.
- **'Eureka' ideas.** They get light-bulb insights, which they are convinced would provide a blanket solution for past misjudgements and mistakes. They set up meetings, make phone calls and send faxes and e-mail toward this end. An example might be attempting to recruit the support of Bill Gates in person to invest in and to save their company from liquidation.
- **The Holy Grail** and other quests. They may become passionate adventurers, heading off to places like Machu Picchu, to white-water raft in New Zealand or to find a guru in India.
- **Sleeplessness.** Their mind is never still, racing thoughts and flights of ideas are the order of the day and night: coupled with enhanced energy this interferes with their sleep pattern, reducing it to one or two hours a night. 'I have too much to do to waste my time sleeping.' This can reach the stage where they literally don't shut an eye for days at a time, in some cases for weeks.
- **Time urgency.** They get impatient at the pace at which things move and want everything to be done yesterday.
- **Short fuse.** There is an anger and irritability when challenged and criticised about their behaviours. They don't suffer 'fools' easily, are impossible to reason with and strenuously resist the restraints of normal life.
- **On the town.** There is a sense that 'I deserve the best'. Money is spent on clothes, presents, nights on the town, champagne, a new car, a brief trip to Rio.
- **God's gift** to women and men. Both sexes who are on the launch pad can become sexually disinhibited and engage in amorous one-night stands.
- **Political incorrectness.** This can range from telling the wrong jokes to the wrong people, making sexual passes at people they would never in their wildest dreams have any interest in, such as their neighbour, an in-law or the boss's wife. This form of promiscuity has no gender difference.

LIFTING OFF INTO ORBIT

The die is cast and is rolling. An unstoppable energetic and chemical shift is underway. Their metabolism is turbocharged and their consciousness is so single-minded, passionate and goal-orientated that it will not be deflected. They feel fantastic and 'over the moon', hence the association with the term 'elation' (which comes from the Latin *efferre* meaning to lift up, inspire with pride, lift the spirits of, or to feel exalted and lofty).

Lift-off is recognised by a total loss of contact with this reality due to the assumption of an alternative persona. This role usually has a grandiose quality to it, giving sufferers a sense of power, success, confidence and a feeling that everything is going really well and that they are in full control. They become super-fixers with God-like powers and believe that they are the custodians of the solutions for which humanity has been waiting — e.g. Third World economic programmes, global conflict resolutions, scientific discoveries and breakthroughs in medical science.

Others believe that they have extraordinary talents in the area of music, acting, film, as yet undiscovered by the entertainment world. Like a good method actor they take on the persona that fits closest to the wildest dreams of their prior personality — then they live this role around the clock. They have entered the megalomaniac stage (from the Greek word *megas*, meaning great or very large).

Lift-Off Symptoms

- **Increasing distance**. The gap widens between their reality and that held by those around them. This gives rise to reciprocal frustration, irritability, angry outbursts and a total breakdown of normal communication and relationships.
- **The loss of a personal censor**. Anything goes: 'I will not be stopped and no-one is going to stand in my way.' There is a refusal to be censored by the outside. Threats such as loss of job, collapse of relationships, suspension of credit and legal interventions all fall on deaf ears.
- **Hostile behaviours**. With the combination of time urgency, grandiosity and their conviction that the end

justifies the means, support is extorted to validate their views, which are patently obvious to others as ludicrous.

- **Conspiracy theories abound.** This provides a logical explanation to them as to why they are not being facilitated with urgent meetings, financial support and public acclaim. 'Those that are not with me are against me.'
- **Hitting the wall.** As in the old proverb, they have given themselves enough rope to hang themselves with and the noose begins to tighten. Spouses, children and friends withdraw. Financial resources dry up and all credibility collapses. Lack of sleep, excessive substance abuse, inadequate diet, erratic routines and emotional turmoil from ongoing conflict begin to take their toll on their energy reserves.
- **Hospitalisation.** Inevitably there comes a time when the long-suffering relatives reach their limit and decide that in the individual's own interest, the best thing that could happen to them is something akin to a shot from a tranquillising gun. There is general agreement that the cycle has to stop. This may mean that they are coerced or involuntarily committed into a psychiatric institution.

RE-ENTRY — CRASH-LANDING — FALLOUT

Energy bankruptcy — metabolically there are not the reserves to deal with the overwhelming demands at this time. The batteries are now flat and biochemically they are in a state of metabolic burn-out. Sleep deprivation, lack of food, substance abuse and the relentless chaotic activity has created a toxic state from which the individual now needs to recuperate.

Psychoactive medication — this is used to bring the manic phase to a close. It does so by slowing the metabolism, reducing the manic thoughts and the hyperactivity. Essentially the initial phases of medication act as sleep therapy. The restoration of sleep reduces the hypersensitivity of the nervous system to the aminergic family of mind-brain chemicals (i.e. adrenaline and serotonin, the struggle-striving hormones). This allows the cholinergic family (i.e. acetylcholine, the hormone of balance and maintenance) to catch up and restore normality. In the words of Shakespeare, 'Sleep is nature's balm.' While medication is essential to end the destructive manic flight, functioning like a pharmacological straightjacket, it creates a state of suspension or twilight zone where normal psychological and emotional responses are slow to return. This phase can be extremely distressing for relatives, particularly children, who find parents zombie-like and unresponsive.

- **Wounded pride**. Pride comes before a fall. A free-falling manic topples from a great height and the impact reflects that fact. As they return to everyday consciousness and their previous identity, they are faced with a scene equivalent to the post-battle scenario. It is similar to a defeated general reflecting on the number of lives needlessly lost and the futility of the cause fought for with such blinkered single-mindedness.

- **Disillusionment**. As the medication is gradually decreased and awareness starts to percolate through, many become deeply depressed by the outlook — making problem-solving an additional overwhelming burden. One of the primary disillusionments is that in spite of their 'great escape', on their return they are still facing the predicament of impending failure from which they took flight — now seriously compounded by the visible debris resulting from the manic episode itself. This can include severed relationships, financial ruin, loss of others' confidence and trust, the jeopardising of a good work record and promotional possibilities. In some cases there are even more serious consequences, such as legal proceedings pending as a result of car accidents, broken contracts, violent behaviour, barring orders, protection orders, paternity suits, all of which demand urgent attention at a time when sufferers are at their lowest.

- **Suicidal thinking**. For some this seems like the only reasonable solution — so great is their shame. 'There is no way out.' Their flight into mania, which was an unconscious effort at a solution, has inevitably created more problems that it has solved. So deep is the feeling of despair, desolation and hopelessness that the pain of it dictates an action which will end it. In this sense it is a form of self-administered euthanasia.

- **The medication seesaw**. Manic patients, having been brought back to consensus reality by high doses of sedative medication may now find themselves — particularly if they are deeply depressed and suicidal — being prescribed psychic energisers (antidepressant medication) to provide a mood elevation. Consequently, the mood will often elevate to such a point that another manic episode is triggered and corrective sedative medication is prescribed to dampen it. This 'relapse' can be a further blow to patient and family, so soon after the manic episode. Alternating mood swings of this kind, highs and lows, can give rise to the diagnosis of a 'bipolar' disorder (manic depression) and the goal becomes one of 'balance' — balancing out the sufferer's mood.

The professional patient — having left hospital, many sufferers become professionally trained *mood watchers*. They may lose their sense of perspective as to what are acceptable normal levels of joy and excitement, or their opposites, having an off day. Juggling doses of medication can become the sole focus of out-patient consultations, reinforcing the notion that 'relapses' are caused purely by 'chemical shifts'. In this way medication is seen as 'corrective'. Unfortunately this balancing act can become a lifelong process. To break this disempowering cycle, psychotherapy is vital to make sense of the underlying inability to deal with failure and to take up the challenge of being ordinary. Locating the primary problem at source — thought — is patently unavoidable if the *cycle of cause and effect* is ever to be broken.

LET'S ASK OUR PANEL OF EXPERTS

Let us bring in our panel and see what they have to say about Julian's manic flight, described in Chapter 3. Since he left the concert in a 'blaze of glory' they have been watching his progress.

Convinced of his brilliance, Julian was driven by the notion that he was 'the one' to bring Messiaen to the concert halls of the world under the guidance of the Archangel Gabriel. In the following days he hounded his agent demanding to know why press conferences, television and radio interviews were not happening now that he was the 'star'. He hit the town in celebration of his success and of his mission. He socialised in fashionable bars and night clubs and entertained lavishly. He dressed flamboyantly, slept infrequently, spent large amounts of money, borrowed extensively and accumulated a group of hangers-on whom he regaled with his grandiose plans. Nightly he partied. His quick wit, charm, high energy and the endless flow of champagne created an ambiance which attracted males and females alike. He exuded a sexual magnetism and had no problem finding willing partners.

He was having the best time of his entire life. He felt his mental faculties had expanded and that he was in touch with otherworldly powers. His mind worked like lightning, guessing what people were thinking and finishing off their sentences. Walking into a room, attention gravitated toward him instantly. With no more than schoolboy French and tourist Italian he laced his dialogue with fanciful superlatives, testing out his fluency on barmen, waitresses and any tourist he happened to encounter.

One night he held a fancy dress party at his apartment. Guests were invited to dress as 'Angels or Transvestites'. Hundreds arrived and the place was packed to capacity. A samba band played enthusiastically to his constant shouts of encouragement. He danced wildly on top of the grand piano, dressed as the Angel Gabriel. With flapping wings he 'flew' from the piano knocking people to the ground as he landed on top of them. He rushed to an open window shouting that he was going to join the gods and play Messiaen in heaven!

As concerned friends pulled him off the window ledge, he became enraged, ripped off his wings and started to kick and punch them — panic broke out. While some people tried to hold him down, others scattered. One of his neighbours, already incensed by the nightly disturbances, loud music and his unwillingness to listen to their objections, finally decided enough was enough — he called the police. Outraged by their intrusion, Julian ordered them out of the apartment. After a series of unheeded cautions and a protracted struggle, they arrested him. He is led away handcuffed, cursing their insubordination. He accuses them of being part of a conspiracy by the Conservatoire to prevent him bringing Messiaen to the masses.

Hours later he finds himself in the nearest psychiatric institution being forcibly injected with medication.

The Panel's View of Julian's Condition

Joe (layperson): 'He's been euphoric for weeks. The concert literally went to his head. For his own sake it's just as well that a stop has been finally put to his gallop.'

Ruth (psychotherapist): 'Julian's been blinded to reality, his thinking world had no room for failure. He was programmed in such a way that anything other than success created a crisis of identity. He must have felt so backed into a corner by his debacle at the Conservatoire in Paris that his mind had to cook the books. His survival literally depended on succeeding at all costs.

'Where did he get all that energy? The speed of his mind was amazing. He was just bursting with brilliance and confidence. What a pity he had to be manic to be like that. Isn't that the attraction of mania, becoming the person you'd most like to be? I've heard many say that they find it so depressing when it burns out. I can see how mania must be so addictive and a difficult pattern of behaviour to give up. It's like an amazing drug.'

Professor Moore (mind-brain specialist): 'The chemistry involved in the genesis of his mania certainly is very interesting. It is extraordinary how the manic flight has parallels with intoxication by recreational drugs such as amphetamine, cocaine and ecstasy. What is remarkable is the fact that the manic chemistry is not artificially created and it builds on itself, gathering momentum as it unfolds.

'It started with his non-acceptance of failure. This mindset created the molecules of adrenaline. Hyperaroused, he went into overdrive, practising all the time — as with all adrenaline states, sleep became a casualty.

'Sleep deprivation plays a huge part in the generation of the manic state. If sleep doesn't happen, the chemistry of the night, acetylcholine-like substances — so vital to balance out the chemistry of the day, i.e. adrenaline-like substances — get eclipsed. In other words, the adrenaline-serotonin family becomes dominant. Now the brain never shuts down. It's in wakeful mode morning, noon and night — no sleep. A never-ending spin cycle of thoughts and the resulting moods — no let up. The result is a major imbalance with serotonin to the fore. The outcome is a certainty — mania! It's like a naturally occurring ecstasy and/or cocaine trip lasting several weeks.

'One can only guess at how much serotonin depletion there must be when it has run its course, as reflected in the burn-out and depression which follows. Like the authors have been saying — the trip has only so much juice. Once the rocket is launched it runs a predictable course — it orbits, re-enters and inevitably crash lands!'

Jackie (energy therapist): 'That fits exactly with what I saw, his sixth chakra (see Appendix) was in overdrive — that's the centre where we create our visions. This provided him with a solution, albeit a delusion, a way of seeing himself as a brilliant, successful pianist. His identity depended on it. Julian's experience at the Conservatoire, where he felt he was no longer in control, was too much for his underdeveloped third chakra. That's the centre of personal power, the place from which we exert influence over our life. If it's not developed we don't have the know-how to manifest our dreams in concrete form. It's for this reason that many people's plans come to nothing.

'During a child's formative years there are three critical developmental tasks from the point of view of the chakra system. They form the bedrock on which the child's personality is based. In the intrauterine period, as well as the first twelve months of life, the child's initial energetic task is to firmly implant in the physical world by developing their first chakra. This means that their physical being makes an energetic commitment to be here.

'With this physical identity in place, the next task is to establish emotional identity which takes place between the ages of twelve and twenty-four months. At this stage they learn how to get their needs met and how to illicit love from others by learning to run energy through their second chakra.

'With these two processes in place the child is poised between the ages of two and three years to acquire the skills needed to effectively control his or her life, achieve things and exert willpower. In this way an ego is formed, at the third chakra. If it's not, then individual autonomy or the ability to separate from the tribe, doesn't kick in. It's about making decisions for yourself and taking risks. The following metaphor is useful: "When your tribe comes to a fork in the road and they all swing right, for your own reasons you may feel it's best to go to the left in spite of the pressure to stay in line."

'In the case of mania, while the first two developmental tasks are complete, the third (ego identity) has not fully matured and grown to its full potential. Even though they have managed to put across a version of themselves as a viable individual, this only lasts as long as certain conditions are met. They can remain confident and sure of themselves only *as long as* they continue to be successful, others approve of them and things keep going their way.

'Any evidence of a potential failure will trigger a crisis of identity. They can just about manage to function without these basics in place in the same way that a mature oak with weak roots can stay upright — but only as long as the weather remains favourable. When they see a threat on the horizon which they lack the skills to respond to, it is then that they move their energy up to the sixth chakra in search of a solution. This is understandable, as their rarefied world of success and ease has up to now given their third chakra little practice in dealing with failure. They are familiar only with the territory of being the best. When reality lets them down, a delusion of continued success is substituted.

'The task of the sixth chakra is to provide us with understandings, insights and beliefs which explain reality to us. The shifting of energy to the sixth, as happened to Julian during his manic flight, provided him with a version of himself of which he approved — at this stage manics are unaware that they have cooked the books. I call it 'vision blindness'. Blind to the realities close at hand, they're like someone who is already talking about the wedding with the person they have just met.'

Patrick (spiritual healer): 'The manic state is so different from the schizophrenic one and yet they're often confused. Unlike mania, schizophrenia has most of the energy concentrated in the seventh (spiritual) chakra. With schizophrenia the most problematic chakra is the first, rather than the third, as in mania. John and Julian's childhoods were, as we've mentioned already, like chalk and cheese. It's important to point out, however, that some manics get so energised that they start to access their seventh. In this way they introduce a spiritual flavour into the delusions created by their sixth. Julian brought in the Archangel Gabriel and this fitted with his dream of 'announcing' or bringing to the world the splendour of Messiaen's music.

'Unlike Julian, Max the rally driver, who the authors wrote about earlier in the chapter, had no 'need' to access the spiritual dimension at the seventh chakra in order to make him feel complete. He had more than enough grandiosity at the level of his sixth. You know what I mean, 'I'm the great businessman' sort of stuff. Julian on the other hand saw himself as being the world's greatest pianist, but also saw himself as having an evangelical role and who better than the Archangel Gabriel?

'This crisis has brought Julian to a fork in the road. He needs to be helped to understand his symptom as a messenger and to use it to throw the focus on how he lives in fear of failure. (See Chapter 3 — I Don't Want to Be Here.) His choice is clear, either continue taking medication for life to prevent a 'relapse' or take the opportunity (an option rarely offered) to be personally involved in the challenging task of learning and transforming oneself — the opportunity to push the envelope a little. Unfortunately long-term medication will paradoxically paralyse his sixth chakra, the very place that can bring him insight. Once Julian has returned to earth, a homeopathic remedy would allow him to stay in balance without his thinking being clouded. Learning how to run his own energy by understanding his chakra system would also help him to help himself.

'As we discussed in the chapter on schizophrenia, psychotherapy is just as important in mania. It helps them understand the role their thoughts had in starting the whole process. It gives them an opportunity to debrief and to cope with the collateral damage they've caused. Did you know that the term psychotherapy is derived from the Latin *psyche* plus *therapiea* meaning soul-attending or soul therapy? His karmic task is to learn to be ordinary and deal with setbacks like the rest of us.'

Dr Henry (psychiatrist): 'It's my opinion that Julian is suffering from a chemical imbalance resulting from a dysfunction in his brain. He's what I would call a manic depressive. Sometimes it's called a bipolar disorder. In other words, he'll experience highs and lows all his life. His first 'low' was when he came back from Paris and now he's experiencing a 'high'. The way he thinks and his lifestyle have nothing to do with the shifts in his chemistry. He is suffering from a disease that requires treatment. Medication is the only thing that will keep him in balance and he will require it for life.'

Dr Clarke (homeopath): 'Balance is the cornerstone of homeopathy but not in the way psychiatry uses the term. Rather than use the same medication to balance all of us, homeopathy would recognise that we each have an individual point of balance within our distinct constitutional nature. Hundreds of these points of balance have been described. We see imbalance as leading to symptoms, either physical, emotional or mental, which are expressed in our own unique way through our personal mannerisms and traits. Each of us has our own way of drifting off-balance. Homeopathic remedies are prescribed from this individualistic perspective, based on the centuries-old truth: *similia, similius curentur,* like cures like.

'While I absolutely accept that major tranquillisers are necessary to dampen down Julian's manic chemistry, he may well have benefited from a remedy in the early stages — for example, when he was feeling a failure and under pressure to succeed. Any later and the imbalance gets too extreme and it has to be handed over to the firefighters — the psychiatrists. However, in his long-term management homeopathy has a place.'

Professor Moore (mind-brain specialist): 'While psychoactive medication unquestionably can bring the manic episode under control, many individuals feel curbed by its long-term use. Many stop taking it for this reason. Inevitably they go high again, since the same mindset is still in place and become chronic revolving-door patients. The real cause of the problem, their thought patterns, never gets addressed. If we were brutally honest we'd have to admit that even if they stay on medication, for many people, their manic episodes keep recurring.

'It is a tragedy that homeopathy has become marginalised from the whole area of madness. A discussion between the two disciplines is long overdue. It doesn't matter to me whether they are called remedies or medicines — as a scientist I'm only interested in what works. Psychoactive medication has the advantage in the manic phase because it's rapidly effective, but it has disadvantages long term because of its numerous and serious side effects. Homeopathy on the other hand is not powerful enough to stop the manic phase, but has the edge long term because it has no side effects. In the world of healing there is no room for exclusivity, professional egotism and pedantic manoeuvrings — the patient comes first.'

CHAPTER 7 — OBSESSIVE-COMPULSIVE DISORDERS

Keynote: Neutralising Wrongdoing

Tommy thinks that if he accidentally brushes against a house-plant on the stairway, he will have to go up and down six times, taking every second step at a time without holding on to the banisters. He does this in order to correct his 'misde-meanour' and thus ensure that his family and girlfriend will be spared from suffering any injury that day.

Ann feels compelled to get in and out of bed exactly fifteen times each night before she can give herself permission to go to sleep. She does the same thing twenty times each morning, to ensure that her husband and children will stay healthy.

If you met Tommy or Ann at work you would never sus-pect that they engage in such extra-ordinary rituals. Welcome to a typical day in the life of an obsessive-compulsive disorder or OCD sufferer! Hollywood highlighted the condition through the character portrayed by Jack Nicholson in the movie *As Good As It Gets*. But Shakespeare was there before him, in the character of Lady Macbeth. 'Out damned spot!' was certainly not an adver-tisement for a washing powder, but the story of a woman over-whelmed by guilt and suffering from this complaint.

All these characters are technically mad because they engage in irrational behaviours, which make absolutely no sense to the watching outsider. However, if you had an under-standing of their mindsets and inner voices, all would be revealed. OCD, in common with all other forms of madness, has its own logic.

Obsession: *is the haunting, possessing and filling of the mind continually and intrusively against their will.*
Compulsion: *is the irresistible impulse to behave in a certain way despite one's conscious intent or wish.*   Oxford Dictionary

PORTRAIT OF AN OBSESSIVE-COMPULSIVE

You feel permanently caught in a web of dread. You fear that you may, for instance, contaminate others with the germs you carry on your hands, in your nose, in your saliva and even on your clothes. You imagine that you have picked these germs up from toilet seats, door handles, money, handshakes etc. and can subsequently pass them on, causing serious illness. With such thoughts in place cleansing rituals evolve. You become obsessed with washing. Avoidance rituals are a compulsion, such as using a handkerchief on a doorknob, turning taps on with your elbows and taking care to avoid body contact at all costs.

Elaborate, inconvenient and time-consuming behaviours fill your days. You might go so far as to believe that, while you may not have AIDS yourself, you are a carrier. Therefore you will take elaborate steps not to contaminate others through sneezing, hand shaking etc. These convictions are to your mind absolute and not open to contradiction.

Other forms of safety-conscious thoughts are common. You may have doubts that electrical and gas appliances have been left on, windows and doors left unlocked and taps running. The list is endless and your *checking behaviours* always need to be repeated. The simple routine of leaving your house for work, or to do a school run, can consume hours of time and become hell for yourself and those around you. The execution of a morning ritual means you have to get up at the crack of dawn. This is incomprehensible to others who cannot appreciate that these rituals must be performed to your satisfaction before you can leave the house. Anyone who lives with an OCD sufferer is a worthy nominee for the Nobel prize for patience!

Sometimes superstitious thoughts predominate. If things are not done in a particular sequence, such as getting out of bed, dressing and walking down stairs in a specified way, you are convinced that there will be disastrous consequences for others. This exaggerated sense of duty and responsibility toward the safety of others can even extend to the notion that you have knocked someone down in your car. This means that you have to drive back over the route any number of times, or frantically phone the local Accident and Emergency Department hoping and praying that an ambulance hasn't attended an accident on your particular stretch of road.

The OCD Mindset — *Written in Stone*

The sinking of the *Titanic* involved many variables, none of which were entirely responsible, but all played a part.

Similarly, the mindset behind OCD is multicausal and incredibly complex.

Any of us in the grip of fear, doubt and mental turmoil can find *comfort and appeasement* in behaviours such as making the garage neat and tidy, cleaning out cupboards, washing floors and generally engaging in tidying and cleansing activities, sometimes for days at a time. The Japanese would call this a Feng Shui of the mind. For someone in the midst of chaos, order can give a psychological foothold from which to operate.

The present-day mindset for some OCD sufferers may have evolved from sexual or physical abuse in childhood, as the child's only way of 'rationalising' the traumatic event. The carrying out of compulsive behaviours helps move them away from fear and chaos, in the direction of control and safety.

One distinct form of OCD, whose rituals are played out entirely at the mental level, involves no external behaviour. Even so, these obsessions can be even more depressing, energy draining and time consuming than other forms. Nonetheless, they still elicit feelings of shame, disgust, anxiety and the same sense of wrongdoing. Suddenly sufferers see horrific, depraved and shocking images in their mind's eye, which can take the form of mutilated bodies, decaying corpses, bestial sexual acts and bloody acts of violence. They may visualise themselves as active players in inappropriate behaviours like blasphemous acts in public places or gang rape.

Such is the lifelike and overwhelming nature of these images and the anxiety they provoke that sufferers urgently need to neutralise them somehow. These emergencies demand complex, often mind-boggling, distracting manoeuvres. Running alternative mental images of a soothing nature, engaging in complicated mathematical calculations and playing mental scrabble affords temporary relief.

Classic Characteristics of the OCD Mindset

- **Focus on wrongdoing**. This reflects a black and white moralistic view of themselves and the world, usually learned within the family home. No shades of grey are tolerated and everything is divided into good and bad, right and wrong.
- **Punishment orientation**. This emerges from such moralistic beginnings. Bad must be punished and good must

be deserved. It is not uncommon for sufferers to have experienced inquisitions held by parents, with the child being treated as a virtual criminal over some minor misdemeanour which another family would ignore. These children's lives became ruled by clauses — shoulds, musts, have-tos and conditions — before they could feel intrinsically good or deserving. Thoughts from an early age might include, 'Have I done the right thing? Am I going to be blamed for something? Will I be punished?' It is difficult for them not to grow into fastidious, rigid, perfectionist, self-critical, over-responsible, guilt-ridden and shameful people. Their life is full of trip wires.

- **Guilt and shame**. A trigger-hair arousal of guilt and shame exists, as does a distorted relationship with pleasure, spontaneity and often sex. Pleasure has to be deserved, earned and is certainly not allowed spontaneously. Every pleasurable experience goes through the filter of good/bad, right/wrong and a detailed internal analysis made of it. Sex is number one on the hit list. Normal exploratory sex acts like masturbation may be interpreted by such a child as being perverted, shameful, sinful and a further example of their flawed make-up.

- **Others-first focus**. A vigilance exists relative to the well-being of others and a heightened sense of responsibility and duty toward them. This others-first focus is ever present and OCD sufferers are always concerned whether they are injuring or harming others. They worry about exposing others to dangers, contaminating food in cooking, or knocking somebody down on the road. This anxiety spreads into their work; for example, an electrician may believe that he has wired a house incorrectly. Others believe they will cause harm by stabbing someone dear to them with a sharp implement, strangling a child in their care or punching someone standing beside them in a bar.

- **Atonement**. Being accustomed to punishment following a 'bad act' as a form of atonement, children become conditioned to penalise themselves. They will automatically devise their own appropriate penance so that the scales are balanced. Some children will say extra prayers, deliberately avoid food they like, try to be extra helpful around the house and promise themselves that they will never ever repeat the behaviour. In this way the guilt subsides and they begin to feel like a 'good child' again.

- **Self-blame**. Where there is any doubt as to the wrongs of a situation, they will automatically assume that they are at fault — this comes from a basic sense of badness or unworthiness within them. This is such a core habit that it seems to cancel out sources of merit that they could draw from, such as achievements in their work and family life.

- **Mistrust of their own perceptions**. 'No, no, that's not what you saw; no, you don't feel angry; no your sister didn't mean it; no that's not what happened; no you have made that up; no you must be dreaming; no your father would never do that. . .' If this is the feedback that a child gets to their experience, they begin to mistrust themselves, presuming others and in particular adults, are always right. When they themselves are adults and there is no monitoring parent present, *they devise checking rituals to decide if their perceptions are right or wrong*, such is their implicit doubt. They need to know if a wrongdoing has occurred and therefore needs atonement. This tragic cycle squeezes out free will, joy, spontaneity and pleasure.

- **An intolerable rise in tension levels** occurs if there is a question of having done wrong. OCD behaviours can be seen as an addiction. Like all addictions they go through a recognisable cycle of feeling the tension rising, doing a certain behaviour that provides the 'fix' and experiencing a temporary relief until the cycle begins again.

- **Secrecy**. Given their sensitivity to guilt and shame and their belief that *others are always right*, as children these individuals are unlikely to report an abusive event and as adults are unlikely to share their inner turmoil with anyone. This fosters a sense of isolation and alienation.

DELUSIONAL THINKING — *COOKING THE BOOKS*

Perhaps one of the most extraordinary aspects of OCD sufferers is their ability to distort reality. Many would be regarded as being psychotic if it were not for the fact that they are so grounded, for most of the time, in the real world.

Take Christopher, for example. A successful architect, married with three children, he believes that as he drives home from work each evening he knocks people down and either injures or kills them. This conviction compels him to retrace his steps and verify whether he has or has not. He will repeat this many times, causing him to get home late.

His architectural abilities are second to none. His ability to work within a budget, to a time frame and to manage site meetings are much admired. Yet the same man, *en route* from his work to his home, doubts his judgement as to whether or not he has knocked someone down! Even in the absence of confirmatory evidence such as somebody walking out in front of the car, the sound of the impact, a body on the road, or the screams of bystanders, he will still 'cook the books'. He remains convinced. Nothing will satisfy him other than going back and checking. The idea of proceeding home with such a doubt on board is too anxiety provoking. As far as he is concerned he is guilty until he has proved himself innocent.

The mystery is: how can a brilliant architect who handles a vast array of sensory input in his work in a confident and competent fashion, doubt his perception in this particular area on a daily basis? If he were to mistrust his perceptions at work to such a degree he would be unemployable.

What is the seed of such delusions? How is it possible to straddle two worlds?

Second Chakra *Sabotage*

Between the ages of twelve and twenty-four months our emotional identity is formed energetically. This is the time when a child begins to make a distinction between self and other — to establish emotional boundaries and to bond with those around them. This is the explorative phase, during which information is *felt*, taken in as a vibration, rather than understood intellectually. The child learns to make distinctions along the pain/pleasure spectrum. It is at this delicate point in the developmental process where duality is first introduced — this/that, either/or, nice/nasty, etc. They acquire the skill of getting their needs met, eliciting endearment from others and actively drawing pleasurable experiences toward themselves. They learn how to avoid pain and to decide whether the world is trustworthy, whether it is a safe place, where their needs and wants will be met.

If sexual abuse is inflicted on children at this stage, the pain/pleasure relationship gets confused and distorted. They may feel intrinsically bad but be unable to understand why. They have a primitive pre-verbal sense that a taboo has been broken. Unable to put words to their feelings, they cannot share their distress. Nobody is confirming for them that something horrendous has happened although their second chakra (see Appendix) is telling them that it has happened. This situation conditions them to mistrust their feelings and their perceptions. Having had their emotional boundary overwhelmed with the invasive adult energy, they are not developmentally equipped for such a charge. Tremendous insecurity and ambivalence set in as they try to 'make sense' of the betrayal. These experiences have a lasting impact and make their full presence felt in adult life.

Guilt is instilled as a conditioned response at this age and becomes incorporated into the developing conscience. It becomes the price that one pays for wrongdoing. (The word 'guilt' derives from Old English origins to mean *crime*, *sin* and *should*.) Once guilt is firmly in place, a manipulative adult can more easily 'have their way' by triggering its arousal. Of all the buttons implanted in childhood, guilt has to be one of the most damaging.

Guilt is a social construction, a taught emotion and a form of social control, particularly employed by the various religions. The Christian churches, particularly the Catholic Church, relied for its maintenance of power on control of the body which was seen as a source of evil, an impediment to salvation. Controlling sexuality was central to this maintenance of power. Shame and guilt around sexual expression was firmly implanted. Sex was seen solely as a means of procreation within the confines of matrimony. Confessing one's sins to a priest in the secrecy of a confessional box were mandatory. There, interrogations took place as to the sexual activities of the mind and body.

As God's delegate, the priest had enormous power because he reminded the penitent of the possibility of eternal damnation in the fires of hell. Even small children, whose right it is to be spontaneous, playful, joyful and orientated toward pleasure, were curtailed and constrained in the name of being a 'good child' — making them more lovable to their parents and ultimately to God. It was traditional that during Lent children would make sacrifices which might include 'giving up sweets'.

Many children grew up in households where pleasure was suspect. It had to be earned and was seen as a 'reward' for helping around the house, doing well at school and obeying their parents at all times. In other words pleasure was conditional and conditioned. If you were 'good' you were allowed it, if you were bad you were punished — pain was inflicted. It is rare to find OCD sufferers who have not had a religious upbringing, or at least one in which puritanical values dominated.

Since guilt goes hand in glove with punishment, in later life the adult with such a compromised second chakra will engage in atonement behaviours of their own design for perceived wrongdoing. Now, whenever their guilt builds to an intolerable level at their second chakra, it is at this point that the sixth chakra *offers the solution* — absolution: a way to neutralise the feeling of wrongdoing.

The function of our sixth chakra is to offer us understandings, insights and beliefs that help us make sense of our world. If OCD sufferers can identify the transgression then they can atone for it. In the absence of a real misdemeanour they invent one. 'I am responsible for carrying a deadly virus. I am responsible for knocking someone down on the side of the road.' They follow this with a *logical* solution. 'I must keep my hands clean.' 'I'd better go back and check for a body on the road.'

The dirty hands and the body are delusions, beliefs in a reality that is not shared by others. By completing the required ritualistic cycle the books are balanced and the guilt can subside. By acting out a ritual selected by their sixth chakra (which is symbolic and archetypal by nature) their tension subsides and they have been returned to the status of 'good' person again. They have done their penance!

The reason why the behaviours of OCD sufferers seem illogical, is that they are disconnected from the present day. They are in fact deep-seated, largely unconscious 'hangovers' from early life. Vigilance about goodness is now a habit, it is in fact an obsession, which on a daily basis is keyed into and old buttons pressed causing the tension to rise. With the delusion in place, a symbolic way of lowering it is created and compulsively re-enacted. How else does it make sense for every door, window, tap, plug, etc. to be repeatedly checked when it is patently obvious in the present that there is no threat and that nobody is going to punish them, even if they do leave a light switch on?

Ann (whom we met at the start of this chapter), a 35-year-old mother of two, in addition to her bed rituals avoids preparing food for anyone outside her immediate family. She is convinced she will contaminate them with the AIDS virus. In spite of testing negatively several times in different laboratories, her doubt persists.

She was raised by strict, conservative, Catholic parents with a distant authoritarian father and a puritanical domineering mother, who ran the household along regimental lines. Everything had to be in its right place. Children were seen and not heard, anything worth doing was worth doing well. It was all work and no play — as a child she did not have much fun. Hanging out and relaxing was for lazy people. 'The idle mind is the devil's playmate.' Punishments for 'bad behaviour' were dished out daily. *Guilt was instilled as a deterrent* and a way of policing the children. Ann, being the eldest, bore the brunt of it.

To secure her parents approval, her policy was to be 'good'. This meant that she had to be watchful that everything she did was perfect and above criticism. Whenever she felt pleasure, side by side with it was the feeling that she was 'bad'. Insidiously, she learned not to trust her normal childhood urges.

Teenage activities such as having boyfriends and going to discos were made a misery for her. Her mother would make her ashamed of her appearance as she prepared to go out. 'Ann, no daughter of mine is going out in public like that. What are those things hanging from your ears? Take that lipstick off, it makes you look like a prostitute.' Ann learned that sexual interactions were synonymous with 'loose morals'. The other dominant theme in the home was 'Always put other people's needs before your own.' She learned to tune out her own needs and wants and to second-guess those of others.

On leaving school she trained as a medical laboratory technician. The laboratory tested for serious life-threatening illnesses such as hepatitis and other infectious diseases. Ann's over-conscientious habits got the better of her. She began to have doubts that she might be mislabelling test tubes and causing mistaken diagnoses and interventions. To allay her fears she began going to work early in the morning when the lab was quiet, to furtively double-check her case load. Within a year this had evolved into full-blown obsessive checking routines. She found it increasingly difficult to leave work and was often to be found working into the small hours. Her stress levels now through the roof, she abandoned her training and took up secretarial work.

Over the years she has tried different medications in varying doses and combinations — they didn't work. She still had the OCD drives. She disliked the fact that the medications made her drowsy and the 'unreal' mood associated with it.

Early in her marriage she believed that while drunk at a Christmas party, she might have had a sexual encounter with her brother-in-law who had a reputation as a philanderer. She was plagued with guilt and shame. Although she'd only danced with him, she was turned on. She worried that this may have led to an inappropriate sexual act, the memory of which the alcohol had blotted out. So little did she trust herself, that she was prepared to believe not only that she had had full sexual intercourse with him, but had also contracted the AIDS virus. From then on she avoided cooking for guests, but since she had to cook for her own family, she came up with a trade-off — the bedtime rituals.

LET'S ASK OUR PANEL OF EXPERTS

Joe (layman): 'Now there's a problem I wouldn't like to have. Can you imagine running my place with all those rituals going on? I'm strapped for time as it is! These people deserve medals just for plodding on as they do. OCD is a no-win condition. You're damned if you do and damned if you don't.'

Dr Henry (psychiatrist): 'Most medics would agree it's one of psychiatry's most crippling conditions. At least if you're 'mad' in some of the other ways we've seen, such as schizophrenia and mania, you're not aware you have a problem. The psychiatric treatment of OCD is notoriously ineffective. Medication rarely controls their symptoms. Since they are a group that are very aware of their distress and the impact it's having on their lives, many become pilgrim patients doing the rounds.'

Ruth (psychotherapist): 'They're a difficult group to help. I've spent consultation after consultation listening to their soul-destroying symptoms and their desperation to find a cure. It's so urgent for them that they don't want to talk about anything else. The condition is so hard-wired, that's because they've such a rigid mindset. Psychotherapy can be invaluable in providing insight and support. It can raise consciousness in such a way that the sufferer can then see the origins of their mindset. With that new understanding, their so called 'illogical' behaviours make some sense. Their delusional thinking can now be related to in a different way. Rather than being seen as pathological, it can be seen as an unconscious solution, an effort to come up with some ritual which allows their deep sense of 'badness' to be temporarily neutralised and the guilt somehow minimised.

'It's particularly effective if it involves the family. Eliciting the understanding of a parent or their partner can be crucial in minimising blame and encouraging acceptance and patience for the sufferer's problem.'

Jackie (energy therapist): 'Children who have been sexually abused or exposed to a strict moral upbringing harbour a deep sense of unworthiness, badness and guilt at a core level which they carry into adult life. Along the spectrum of good to bad, once they recognise themselves as being bad, they feel compelled by the tension which that very thought creates to prove to themselves that they are good. Since they can't travel back to their childhood to undo the 'wrong', they find a dilemma in their present life which has the same aroma and covers the same territory. To fulfil the atonement theme, they need to mimic the original acts and recreate the same emotional flavour.

'They do this by projecting a belief from their sixth chakra that they are contaminated with germs, have injured somebody or have put someone in danger. To them this projection is a truth which they have to act on, for the best possible reasons, to protect others. The sixth chakra then contrives a symbolic undoing ritual which absolves them of guilt. In this way an opportunity has been created to relive the experience and at the same time to solve the dilemma.

'Psychotherapy should also include energetic healing of the second chakra. During the emotional releases which inevitably occur during this work, an unintegrated past experience can be encountered. This is where a past trauma has been buried in the unconscious mind where it festers causing endless surface problems.

'I worked with a client called Sandra who exemplifies this, it was only when she made the buried trauma conscious did she begin to heal. She was a 35-year-old mother of two who was married to a farmer and she had been obsessively hand washing from the age of thirteen. In addition, she repeatedly machine-washed bed linen, underclothing and nightdresses. If they weren't cleaned to her satisfaction she would hand scrub them. This practice of washing and re-washing consumed most of her spare time. She might hand-wash fifty to sixty times a day! Since she was a teenager she had been either prescribed psychoactive medication or involved in behavioural modification programmes — to no avail.

'Early on in her marriage there were sexual problems. She discouraged sexual touching by her husband and intermittently suffered from vaginismus — that's when the vagina unconsciously says 'no'. The arrival of her children put her under time pressure. Not enough time to satisfy her compulsion to wash. In spite of rising tension she somehow managed to cope.

'Things came to a head when her husband bought a new farm. She had always worked with him, but now the increasing demands of the farm and her obsession were in conflict. Her anxiety levels escalated and she found herself needing to spend more time washing. She became depressed and saw no way out of her dilemma. The more she tried to stop her compulsion, the more stress she experienced.

'In our sessions it emerged that Sandra's father, following the death of her mother when she was five, started sexually abusing her — a daily occurrence. It continued until he began another relationship and remarried. She was then aged seven. While I was doing energy work on her second chakra she suddenly had an emotional release — she cried and cried and cried. Later she was able to put images with the emotions that were released.

'She remembered vividly getting out of bed after her father had left her bedroom and repeatedly scrubbing her hands and body while showering. In later sessions she got more in touch with her feelings of anger, guilt and shame. She worked through her deep sense of betrayal by her father, who had wilfully exploited her at such a vulnerable stage of her life when her mother had died. All this was locked up as energy complexes within her second chakra.

'She mourned the loss of her childhood and her compromised sexuality, realising that during her teenage years she had been socially withdrawn, unenthusiastic about school and avoided contact with boys. Her husband was her first and only boyfriend and she described the relationship as based on friendship more than anything else, with little sexual attraction on her part.

'She realised that although she was an innocent party she had taken on the guilt and shame for the abuse. In addition she felt her body was soiled and dirty. As a result she felt an irresistible urge to wash and clean. When she had actually made the link between her obsession and the sexual abuse, she was able to see that the repeated washing represented, in symbolic terms, a cleansing process. The need to wash became less and less.

'Following these insights and with her new-found feeling of control and confidence, I encouraged her to tell her husband about the abuse. To her relief he was both understanding and compassionate. For the first time he was able to make sense of her obsessive behaviour and her avoidance of sexual intimacy. This story has a nice ending. Sandra actually managed to come out from under the rock of her past hurts and rebuild her life — a new one.

'It's important to say that not all OCD sufferers have been sexually abused or vice versa. Those who haven't been abused usually have the background of rigid moralistic mindsets in the family home. I am currently seeing a sixteen-year-old boy, an only child whose parents have 'right and wrong' rules about everything — tidiness, cleanliness, punctuality and socialising. From his earliest memories he remembered being castigated and ridiculed if things weren't done in a 'certain way'. He 'has to' have his uniform laid out and ready the night before, be in bed at a certain time, change immediately and complete his home-work on returning from school.

'There are no exceptions to these rules. Strict codes of etiquette apply at the dining table and when visitors came to the house. Spontaneity is discouraged and 'there is a right way of doing everything'. After years of being raised under this regime he now becomes seriously distressed if anything prevents him from performing these learned rituals. He feels he is not a 'good' person and at times will inflict punishment by mutilating himself as a form of atonement. He actually cuts the inside of both his arms with a razor blade, which releases the pent-up tension.

'There's another group who may have come from relaxed families but who nonetheless develop ritualistic strategies which they would only use during an emotional crisis. They're like a comfort blanket. They use them as a way of controlling the feelings of chaos inside. Ritualistic and perfectionist behaviour can give a sense of order and predictability and are grounding for the individual. In this way, for example, during such times as bereavement, divorce, financial pressure and examinations, many find comfort in these routines.'

Patrick (spiritual healer): 'I agree with everything that's been said, OCD is a very dispiriting condition. It's all-consuming and it doesn't give free will much of a look in. Every neuron is squeezed trying to keep the show on the road. Since it's always at the forefront of a sufferer's mind and can't be suspended for a minute, standing back and taking the witness position is almost an impossibility. That's why it's difficult for them to engage fully in psychotherapy, as their attempts to make changes are constantly sabotaged by the overriding demands of their OCD drives.

'This sabotage creates split intention. The conscious mind wants to get better, while the unconscious wants to maintain the status quo until it's satisfied that the books are finally balanced. These two parts of their mind are like ships in the night passing each other in opposite directions. That's why making them aware of the genesis and impact of their rigid mindsets, whether they evolved from an unresolved traumatic experience or not, is critical — to make the unconscious drive conscious.

' 'Badness' or wrongdoing has been taken in at the level of their second chakra, either because they were abused or have felt, due to their belief system, that they did something wrong. The sixth chakra steps in, attempting to solve the problem, to make them 'good' again. Particularly if there's no memory of this wound, the sixth blames the wounded individual for having caused it. A judgement is passed that atonement needs to be made and it decides how. It conjures up a transgression, like knocking someone down, which they have to take the responsibility for sorting out. The wrongdoing which it conjures up becomes the obsession and the method of neutralising it becomes the compulsion.

'The actual truth of the situation, which is not being fully appreciated by the sixth chakra, is that no wrongdoing ever occurred, no atonement was ever needed and they never were intrinsically worthless or bad. This is a universal truth that applies to all of us, that we are intrinsically good, that love is a constant and does not need to be earned. The problem is that if their heart chakra isn't primed from an early age to receive love unconditionally, they can't express it to themselves without putting conditions on it either.

'Compassion toward themselves is the only means by which their reality can be permanently changed. The very life-force itself which runs through all of us is an expression of love and the divine. In karmic terms the function of their obsession is to reawaken them to their own divinity, release their pain, forgive themselves and regain a sense of goodness.'

Professor Moore (mind-brain specialist): 'The chemistry of OCD is unknown territory. It's such a mixed picture. One minute they're running high levels of adrenaline, which is then released by the ritual, leaving them feeling momentarily calm again. It seems like they can be both mad and sane at the same time.

'Christopher, the architect, is a perfect example. As he's leaving work to go home, the security man saying 'Good evening' to him couldn't be saying it to a saner person. Yet twenty minutes later he's looking for bodies on the road — mad! Likewise when he gets home his wife and children greet someone as normal as you or I. That's why medication is generally so unsuccessful, because the thoughts and the chemistry are constantly shifting, along the spectrum of safety to danger.

'If you could actually isolate the chemistry of an OCD sufferer in full flight and inject it into someone else, the symptoms wouldn't be replicated. The molecules alone aren't enough. You need the obsessional thinking pattern in order to manifest the chemistry. Thoughts are causal, even if they're not conscious — the chemistry, which generates the symptoms, is the effect.'

Dr Clarke (homeopath): 'Scientists know only a tiny fraction of what's going on. Scientists don't actually 'discover' things. They uncover what is being expressed within the laws of nature and 'invent' ways to work with them. It's a bit like that for the OCD sufferer. They have to learn to take advantage of the natural pathways which are in place within all of us. To uncover for example the innate power of compassion and self-love.

'OCD reflects a state of imbalance within an individual's constitution or nature. The vibrational flow of the life-force is disrupted in some people by the rigidity of the parental value system, by specific traumas in childhood and in others by stressful present-day situations. These impressions are expressed in different ways and are recognisable to a homeopath as definable 'states' each treatable by a specific remedy. The key to finding the one single remedy that will restore balance and health in each individual's state, is the one single remedy that matches most closely all the symptoms being felt and displayed on the physical, emotional and mental levels.

'**Arsenicum**, for example, manifests as an overwhelming state of anxiety, insecurity and restlessness which leads to a picture of constant worry, movement and checking. The well-being of the family is a grave concern and they are excessively particular or fastidious about details, their state of health and the presence of germs. It is a major remedy for habitual hand washing. This remedy may suit Sandra. **Syphilinum** is another handwashing and checking remedy.

'**Nux Vomica** would be good for somebody like Christopher who has an exacting nature, likes to be in control and who, when pressured, will feel the need to check and recheck that things are done properly. His compulsion to check whether he has knocked someone down can point to this state.'

CHAPTER 8 — DEPRESSION

Keynote: Dis-Illusionment

Depression is common. At one time or another all of us have experienced it. So, what is it?

We know that it is dramatically different to schizophrenia and mania, both of which fit our usual image of madness. It is a source of much common unhappiness. It can lead to suicide and even murder. How often do you hear of the mother or father who, unable to cope with life, drives the car with their children on board off a pier, drowning everyone? Is this not a form of madness?

Those who experience schizophrenia and mania (psychosis) are definitely in a world of their own and not accessible, as we have seen. Depression is different in that sufferers are not out of reach — they share the same reality as the rest of us. However, a small number can get so deep into depression that they can develop beliefs that are psychotic; they may be convinced, for example, that their body is rotting away and that nothing can stop it happening.

Other fundamental differences between people suffering from depression and those with schizophrenia and mania include their ability to hold down jobs, engage in family life and generally put on a convincing social front. Sometimes this façade fools others so effectively that relatives are devastated by the extent of the deception. We have all heard the stories of how a person has left, for example, a business meeting and was found later in an isolated area, gassed in their car. Alternatively, cases such as the person who, under the guise of a weekend away, shopping or visiting friends, was found overdosed in a hotel room — seemingly 'normal' right up to the end.

What unites all those who experience these psychological distresses is fear. The schizophrenic is afraid of the harshness of this world. The manic fears failure and loss of face. The depressive is afraid that the present will continue indefinitely and that there is nothing they can do about it. This state is also shared by the burnt-out manic who has hit rock bottom. As well as having fear in common, none of them want to continue interfacing with the life they have. 'I don't want to be here.'

Chronic states, be they physical or mental, can be travelling companions of depression. The notion that you are more than likely going to have as much pain and discomfort tomorrow and in the future is depressing stuff. Severe arthritis and other degenerative conditions take a heavy toll. Accepting the constant presence of fear in spite of your best efforts to reduce it, just like Mary, is hard work. Many of those suffering from panic attacks and post-traumatic stress disorder eventually get depressed. Many of the painful inevitabilities of life, such as the death of loved ones, ageing, sickness, broken hearts and illness, are extremely dis-illusioning.

Coupled with the fear in depression is self-loathing, one of the most oppressive and soul destroying of experiences. If we feel we cannot overcome our difficulties, we are conditioned to blame ourselves and loathe what we have become. After all, depression is not on society's list of admirable qualities.

LIFE IS NO LONGER DESIRABLE

YOU ARE WHAT YOUR DEEP DRIVING DESIRE IS.
AS YOUR DESIRE IS, SO IS YOUR WILL.
AS YOUR WILL IS, SO IS YOUR DEED.
AS YOUR DEED IS, SO IS YOUR DESTINY.

UPANISHADS

Depression is best understood as a disorder of desire and will. It is human nature to have desires. To wish, want and hope to have our needs met. To dwell on the future, to plan and to expect certain outcomes and not others. Anticipation gives us a sense of order and control as we try to steer ourselves toward pleasure, safety and security and away from pain, fear or danger. Doesn't every child like to believe that when they are grown-ups they will be successful, contented, loved and secure? It is our game-plan. From an early age we 'look forward' — to Santa coming, to being popular at school, to getting on a team, passing our exams, finding a job and earning our own money, falling in love, having a family and a good lifestyle.

Generally we desire happiness and a safe, easy passage through life and it is this game plan that keeps us motivated and provides us with enough willpower to continue. If it lets us down, if things do not pan out as we had hoped, then there is a sense of loss as our dream dies — as if we have been robbed or something concrete has been taken away from us. In fact it is our *illusion* of an uninterruptedly rosy future that has been removed. So our sense of loss is very real and as much a bereavement as any other.

Alternative and far less desirable future scenarios than those we had planned now confront us. Who allows for rejection, exam failures, being passed over for promotions, infertility, bad investments, problematic children, disability, ageing or loneliness? Unprepared and *dis-illusioned*, we can no longer find within us the desire or the will to engage with such futures. In shock, we wonder what happened to the game plan.

The five classic stages of grief and bereavement unfold within us:

1. 'Could this really be happening to me?' — *denial*
2. 'It's so unfair, I don't deserve this!' — *anger*
3. 'I'll work harder, I'll make it happen.' — *bargaining*
4. 'I give up, I'm not playing the game anymore, what's the use?' — *depression*
5. We hope this unpleasantness will disappear and our reality improves. If it doesn't, we are challenged to get on with the difficult business of living out a future we hadn't planned. — *acceptance*

Across the spectrum of depression there are degrees of severity, in the same way that a swimming pool has a deep and a shallow end. The short term, less intense variety which we all know well is often remedied by strategies in our own personal DIY kit — a holiday, a career break or some 'retail' therapy. Alternatively, we might try distracting ourselves with a new toy such as a car, an extension on the house or a new romance. Others turn to their favourite chemical, such as alcohol or other recreational drugs such as cocaine and ecstasy. Many approach their GP for prescribed versions to give them a 'lift'. Solutions emerge, we find a way round the obstacle, we construct a new game plan and the desire to go on again is rekindled.

Unless we complete these stages and reach acceptance, we are paralysed relative to the future. Until 'desire' and with it 'will', return, there is a sense of being immobilised, demotivated and confused. We are reluctant to go forward and look instead to the past, ruminating over mistakes, cataloguing our worthlessness. Recoiling from what reality has presented us with, without answers and full of guilt and shame, we don't know how to proceed. What do we do when we are enveloped by the fog of confusion?

Feeling too bewildered and helpless to act, we withdraw our will and our energy and feel little incentive to engage with the outside world. Movement slows down, we distance ourselves from loved ones — many find it hard even to get out of bed and cope with the basics of living. Simple tasks such as washing, dressing, preparing food and facing the public take on mammoth proportions.

Too Many Names

Returning to the deep end of our spectrum, it is a misnomer to classify those with severe depression in medical terms such as 'clinical', 'chemical', 'reactive' or 'endogenous'. Anything diagnosed by a doctor, is 'clinical'. This term tells us nothing about the depression itself.

All depression is 'chemical' as is every other emotional state such as fear, anger, love and joy. The dis-illusioned, demotivated, hopeless and paralysed state associated with depression is created by chemical shifts secondary to our consciousness. *So ultimately it is our own perceptions, thoughts and beliefs which lead to such states or ways of being, rather than the other way round.*

Within this understanding, all depression is 'endogenous' (generated from within), even if there is some external event such as a death or disappointment, which we are 'reacting' to.

The packaging or branding of such familiar and ordinary emotions through the use of medical labels has the effect of removing them from such common everyday experiences as grief and loss, dis-illusionment, frustration and unhappiness. These more realistic descriptions point to origins in terms of what the mind has perceived and with which it is dealing. They suggest solutions, although not always ones that can be implemented without societal overhaul on a grand scale. For example, lack of resources can make for less manoeuvrability and control over one's future. The poverty trap, meaningless jobs, dysfunctional relationships and harsh living conditions are factors over which many have little influence.

The *medicalisation* of these problems of living as 'chemical' depression has undoubtedly held back major transformational change in terms of socially-oriented legislation and ultimately the distribution of all kinds of resources. The medical profession has inadvertently allowed itself to be politically manipulated and misused. As a result it has lost its social voice, its role as a witness to the mores of society and its moral standing.

There is many a 'chemical' depression that a lottery win, a proper home, a job or a divorce would solve instantaneously! In the same way, the implications of telling a depressed individual that they have a chemical imbalance which may be *lifelong*, requiring the long-term use of medication and intermittent hospitalisation, must be akin to the diagnosis of an incurable cancer. Is this bleak scenario a source of suicide itself?

VISIBLE AND INVISIBLE DEPRESSION

Some episodes of depression follow events and our reaction to them of which we are well aware, such as a broken romance or work difficulties. The initial stimulus is visible and it is clear we are reacting to it. Others, those at the deep end of the pool or the severe end of the spectrum of depression, are often stimulated by a source which is invisible to us. They can be multilayered in their formation. Many individuals have experienced deep hurts and wounds from very early in their lives, which remain unhealed and buried and which have never been verbalised. These can range from childhood abandonment to sexual abuse, emotional deprivation or a dysfunctional family life. In such cases, a present-day setback may trigger off past emotional traumas and as they begin to resurface, the upset they cause seems out of proportion to the current stimulus. There seems to be no rhyme or reason for the depth of the response.

The medicalisation and pharmaceutical treatment of such cases passes up a valuable opportunity — which counselling and psychotherapy can provide — to permanently heal such old wounds. It is common for clients who have been treated for years with antidepressants to have been harbouring extensive emotional pain such as childhood abuse. These buried, unacknowledged complexes or energy vortices — which by definition are out of awareness and unconscious and never expressed, processed or worked through — can be called *'unintegrated experiences'*. Vast amounts of energy are haemorrhaged into them, thereby holding back personal growth and normal psychological and emotional development.

SPIRITUAL DEPRESSION

In the middle of the road of my life, I awoke in a dark wood, where the true way was wholly lost.   Dante

Central to spiritual depression is a loss of meaning and life-purpose. Life is 'futile'. The questions 'Why?' and 'What for?' occupy the mind. There is a sense of merely going through the motions of living. Suffering individuals feel dead to themselves and dead to the world. Everything is stripped bare, they stand naked as if on a stage without props or a part to play. They have lost the plot and can find no framework within which to live. The future seems irrelevant and the past a waste of time. This state is truly the 'dark night of the soul'.

Appeals to sufferers to 'make an effort' and 'pull themselves together', are not just useless, but further alienating. The will is paralysed, just as an arm may be paralysed at the physical level. Would you tell such a person to make more effort? Would they then be able to do so? On the contrary, admonishment, advice, platitudes, guilt trips and threats have as much value as flogging a dead horse. This approach adds to the damage. The implied criticism is instantly internalised and used as another weapon against the self. As the self-loathing mounts, many sufferers may actually take seriously the notion of killing themselves.

'I don't want to be here.' All they can see is a black hole. They want to recoil from the world, batten down the hatches, retreat, crawl into their shell and disconnect. If spiritual depression is found in all cultures and in all historical epochs, to what is it trying to draw our attention? Could it be that it is an unconscious attempt to unclutter the mind, by stripping away distractions in order to face their own 'demons'? To reflect on whatever it is that stands between them and peace of mind and a spiritual connection.

In modern society there is little time for personal reflection. Private time out, time actually spent on one's own is not valued enough and is rarely seen as healing. Our personal needs get squeezed out by the whirlpool of work thoughts, money thoughts, traffic thoughts, household thoughts, relationship thoughts, social and leisure thoughts, media thoughts, sitcom thoughts and whatever thoughts are necessary to be a part of this increasingly amorphous mass known as the human 'race'. *Where is the space for personal intimacy and soul thoughts?* This alienated state is summed up by Leonard Cohen:

> THE BLIZZARD OF THE WORLD
> HAS CROSSED THE THRESHOLD
> AND IT HAS OVERTURNED
> THE ORDER OF THE SOUL.

Increasingly, it seems as if we are propelled from behind, to keep moving forward, to stay engaged, not to fall back and to keep the juggling act going. We are like mice on a moving treadmill. The paradox is that in depression, either falling off or willingly stepping off the treadmill is precisely what is needed. But it is extremely difficult in our *quick-fix, feel-good* culture. There is little permission or validation for disengaging from society for a period. The conditioning against doing so is reflected in the stigma and shame sufferers feel on admitting they have been depressed. This is not an experience that those taking time out after a bypass or a slipped disc have to deal with.

We need to be offered the support and given the guidance to see our depressed state as a natural phenomenon, arising with due cause and requiring serious appraisal. Much like the oil indicator light in the car, depression can be seen as a need for urgent attention, a symptom of a troubled soul and as a signal to get off the treadmill and invest time in inner reflection. Such 'soul pain' needs space to process itself.

By medicalising this stage and using the popular psychic energisers such as Prozac, Efexor and its cousins, we may find ourselves jump-started prematurely back into action. With this boost we may be able to interface again with the details of our life, but it is at the cost of awareness as *the messenger is not afforded a listening space.* There has been insufficient time for new insights or new skills to be gained. Inevitably 'relapse' is on the cards.

A point frequently forgotten is that long-term use of medication creates dependency. The body's own mechanisms of producing the necessary chemicals get turned off by the presence of an artificial source. For example, what about the commonest cause of infertility — the long-term use of the contraceptive pill. Why is this? It is because the ovaries literally 'forget' how to produce eggs!

By understanding the 'checks and balances' in the world of the body's biochemical system, the cycles depressives go through become understandable. If the patient suddenly stops taking their medication, there is a gap in production of the 'feel-good' hormones such as serotonin. This depressed mood can be interpreted as a relapse. In fact, it is withdrawal. Medication is invariably restarted.

A TYPICAL DAY IN CARMEL'S LIFE

'Oh my god, he's awake again. Will it ever stop? I haven't had more than three hours uninterrupted sleep since Luke was born. He's a year old, you'd think he'd have settled by now. I didn't realise I was living with a deaf man until the kids arrived! Another day of feeling wiped out. How will I get around the shops with the pair of them hanging on to me? At least Jack is finally walking, I won't have to carry him.'

Later in the supermarket at the checkout. . .

'Cash or visa?'

'Cash? Wouldn't I love to have some cash, I'd be on the first plane to the Bahamas. This Prozac sure ain't working. I didn't bargain for it all being so difficult. When this is done with I'll treat myself to a Danish in Joe's.'

'How are things Carmel?' Joe asks jovially.

'How long have you got? I'm still not getting a wink of sleep with the little one. There's days when I really wish I was back working full-time. I feel much better when I'm at work.'

'Sounds like you need to get a good child-minder so you can get back out there.'

'Wouldn't I love to, but Daniel is out of the old mould and wants to have them 'mothered' properly. If he only knew! I've had visions of throwing Luke out the window. Anyway Joe, give me a nice Danish and I might get through the morning.'

Back at home, with the children watching cartoons, Carmel stares vacantly out the window:

'There's no way I'm going to have the energy to pack the dishwasher. I just can't go on with this sham, keeping up appearances,

smiling at the neighbours and keeping my mother happy. Will she ever get off my case? She's been making me feel really guilty about wanting to go back to full-time. "Children need their mothers for the first five years and you don't exactly need the money." I thought I could at least rely on her to understand and give me more of a hand. What I wouldn't give for a day in town on my own! I can't remember when I last got my hair done. It's all so depressing. If only there was a way out.

'Daniel's not the worst, he knows I'm having a tough time of it. Like me he wonders why the antidepressants aren't working. This all only started three months ago so I know it's not baby blues.

'I never thought I'd feel so trapped. They never told us about this one in school. Funny, after all the running around having a great time, all I thought I needed was a nice marriage and children. Now I have them. So why do I hate my life? All my friends seem to be able to cope, I don't hear them bitching about it. What's the matter with me then?

'I wish there was somebody I could talk to. My doctor's nice, but he doesn't really understand how awful I feel. He genuinely thinks the tablets are going to work. If only. . .'

LET'S ASK OUR PANEL OF EXPERTS

Two months later, the panel watch as Carmel has her stomach pumped out in an Accident and Emergency Department following an overdose.

Dr Henry (psychiatrist): gives his diagnosis. 'She's suffering from endogenous depression and was obviously suicidal. Her doctor should have increased the medication and if that didn't work had her admitted to hospital for a course of electric shock treatment.'

Ruth (psychotherapist): disagrees, 'I never bought that endogenous label, that there is no *known* cause. It's ridiculous to put it all down to chemistry. It's such a blanket diagnosis and it turns people into chemical cripples. If you take thought, mindset, emotions and living circumstances out of the equation, you're removing everything personal that causes it and you're merely focussing on the effects. Just because the underlying reasons may not be obvious, or can't be verbalised, doesn't mean they're not there. Emotional pain can be very deep and subtle and depression can mask it, sometimes for years.'

Jackie (energy therapist): gives her opinion. 'I've seen people who've had childhoods of terrible abuse. Their energy field contains complexes of energy which have never been processed or worked through. The experiences are totally outside of their awareness and can remain buried in their unconscious for years. The big problem is that vast amounts of energy, which should be available for personal growth, get haemorrhaged in order to keep them buried, kept safely underground. *Out of sight out of mind.*

'They're just too disturbing to be looked at and experienced. The consequences are much too overwhelming for them. Who wants to be aware that their father abused them at a young age? We don't have such protective defences for nothing. I see none of those buried traumas in Carmel's energy field. Her childhood was as normal as the rest of us, although her mother was a bit old-fashioned.'

Patrick (spiritual healer): 'If you want a label for what's wrong with Carmel, I can give you one, but it's not one you'll find in the textbooks. It's a soul cry, a *spiritual depression*. This happens when the *game plan* lets us down. Carmel over-invested in the *happy family* thing to the extent that she forgot about her own needs and desires. Three years later she wakes up to find her life empty, with a sense that something is missing and yearning for more.

'She's feeling just like Dante said, "In the middle of the road of my life, I awoke in a dark wood, where the true way was wholly lost." She is being challenged to reconnect with herself and free herself from her past conditioning. Carmel is facing a predicament which is the result of past soul-life experiences and a karma which says that she does not have the power to influence her own life effectively.'

Jackie (energy therapist): 'Carmel's energy system reflects this karma. She's running little or no energy through her chakra system (see Appendix). This is why she is so exhausted all the time and has no enthusiasm for life. She's been having that feeling that there's a glass pane between her and the world. It's as if she's been on the outside looking in. Her third chakra, the one that gives her personal power, is immobilised. This is why she feels so helpless to act. Her sixth is giving her third the message that 'you don't have the power to change things'. Carmel has yet to learn that this is not true. In karmic terms she's at a major crossroads. The reason she feels so abandoned, disconnected and alienated from everything around her and in particular her soul, is that her seventh chakra is giving its energy to the sixth. That's why spiritual depression is such a good name.'

Ruth (psychotherapist): 'The helpless feeling that she is experiencing is well known as a pattern of behaviour found in many depressed people. Many have an overwhelming feeling of losing control over events. The belief that 'my actions are futile' can be imprinted following a series of experiences, perhaps over an entire childhood, during which *mastery* was not achieved.

'For Carmel, the empowering experience of being her own person and doing what was good for her was denied, given the role modelling she had from her mother. There were more "have-tos" than "want-tos" in her upbringing. Effective psychotherapy would encourage her to put her own needs first and to go with her inner knowing. In short — to turn "I can't" into "I can".'

Professor Moore (mind-brain specialist): 'Helplessness is actually an identifiable chemical state which predominates in depression. When the mind-brain perceives that you are overwhelmed and have lost control, a protective chemical mechanism kicks in. Your system decides, in your best interest, to accept defeat and not waste any more energy fighting a battle you can't win. All the other "action" hormone production, of substances such as adrenaline and serotonin, is put on hold.

'The chemistry of withdrawal and hibernation, predominantly cortisol (also called hydrocortisone), now takes over. "I just want to stay in bed and cover my head." "I can't" creates powerful chemistry. It's as if the body is insisting we recognise that we can only take so much. It's asking us — just like a heart attack does — to slow down, withdraw and reflect. What a pity it's not seen like this by society. Life is just moving too fast nowadays to take time out and read the omens.

'Anti-depressant medications are mood-altering in their action. While the individual may feel better, their ideas which caused the depression in the first place, go unchanged. As long as the "feel-good" experience is maintained everybody is happy. The problem is that because the system gets used to the medication, the effects wear off — back come the same old thoughts. The depressed mood deepens and the medication is increased. Eventually, after trials of different medication, in various combinations and doses, the depression inevitably persists.

The body's ability to manufacture its own anti-depressant chemicals, like serotonin, has become compromised. Now we have a drug-induced depression that has been chemically created.'

Dr Clarke (homeopath): 'Depression is a time for soul-searching. It's a wake up call — a time for reflection and stock-taking. This can be a lonely business and the biggest dis-illusionment for sufferers is feeling that they are not supported by anything "out there". The reality is that the life-force is always taking care of us — a connection to it is like a muscle, it needs to be used or it atrophies. Many look around for support from it when times are hardest —when they don't find it they believe this spiritual force doesn't exist. Ironically, depression points the way to a state where full expression of the life-force becomes compromised.

'Homeopathy is a science which attempts to redress this unhealthy situation. It dissolves the blocks to the flow of energy left by traumatic or stressful experiences — like removing rocks which are interrupting the flow of a river. In this way the life-force or "chi", is free to express itself. Homeopathy has this in common with other energetic healing approaches such as bioenergy and acupuncture (which directly target the energetic system) and psychotherapy which changes thought impulses.

'There are a number of constitutional remedies which can address the imbalance seen in the depressed state. In those who are feeling overwhelmed with life's responsibilities, who have tried their best and find it's still not enough, **Calcarea** is indicated. When the loss of a loved one, as in death or the break-up of a relationship, leads to an overwhelming sense of sadness, **Ignatia** has a place. Some depressed states are dominated by remorse, guilt and ruminations over past painful memories with disillusionment and disappointment over the breaking of trust — they respond to a **Natrum** remedy.

'Carmel's state reflects how we all have a quota system. How far we can be pushed, how many energy drains we can handle, how many disappointments we can sustain, how much sleep we need, how much does life have to unfold as we think it should? How many of all these things does it take to accumulate, and then start pushing us over, off balance into the territory of despair, dis-illusionment and depression?

'For Carmel and her state of depletion, resentment and suicidal attempt, I would consider first **Nitric Acidium** to help her build up her strength and diffuse the bitterness. Next I would consider **Aurum Metallicum**. She had the kind of childhood where love was only forthcoming when she pleased her parents. She had a lot of bottled-up anger and resented the fact that she was so trapped. Like many Aurums she kept up the façade until the end. Aurum is used in the darkest, bleakest, all consuming states where the black cloud descends and engulfs the individual, where life is no longer worth living and suicide is contemplated. "I don't want to be here." **Ammonium Carbonicum** might also fit.

'For states of depression that are mild, many naturopaths might use the herbal preparation Hypericum (or St John's Wort). While it can be effective, a homeopathic remedy has the advantage of working at the level of the energy field, which herbal preparations do not, and in the long run, if matched correctly with each individual's constitutional state, act at a deeper level.'

Patrick (spiritual healer): 'Had she succeeded in taking her own life, she would have missed an opportunity to learn to be effective and to influence her life to move in the direction she wants it to. She is under the false impression that there is nothing she can do about her situation — her karma, or conditioning, is telling her so. If ever there was a place for psychotherapy this is it. It would throw the focus on Carmel's soul needs and how to identify and meet them. Transcending her karma would involve acquiring the personal power skills of the third chakra, in other words learning to assert herself, to stop being a people-pleaser and to realise that she can write her own script.

'I would have one question for her to answer — how can she best serve the needs of her soul, since she is here for that purpose. Once she commits to that task, she would find that a whole stream of life-supporting events will move in her favour. That's what Providence means, the life-force taking care of us.

I believe that what lies at the heart of depression is that the depressed patient believes or has learned that he cannot control those elements of his life that relieve suffering, bring gratification or provide nurture — in short, he believes that he is helpless.   Martin Seligman

CHAPTER 9 — PANIC ATTACKS

Keynote: Red Alert!

Oh my God, I've got to get some air!

'Excuse me! Excuse me! Please get out of my way, I need to get off. Will somebody please pull the cord! Pull the cord! Pull it! Quick, I've got to get off this train, I'm dying. I'm suffocating!'

Jesus, I'll have to do it myself. There it is. What'll I use to break the glass? I know, my shoe! Crash!

'Why did you pull the cord Miss?' asks the driver gently. 'Are you OK?'

'No, I'm dying,' squawks Mary, still clutching her shoe, gasping and choking. 'I can't breathe in here. Please get me off the train.'

An hour later Mary is in the Accident and Emergency Department of Charing Cross Hospital.

'What do you mean everything is OK doctor? It couldn't be, I nearly stopped breathing and my heart was jumping out of my chest. You're obviously missing something, I know something's terribly wrong.'

'No Mary, everything's checked out fine. All you've had is a panic attack and it's over now. Take a seat and we'll order a taxi to get you back to your hotel.'

All! Did he say 'all'? I thought my throat was blocked and my heart was flying and he's telling me I'm fine! What did he give me Valium for? Does he think I imagined it? If that's the case I must be going mad.

Mary has just survived her first panic attack. In the taxi, replaying the drama of the morning, she tries to make sense of it. Questions and images race through her mind.

What came over me? Something weird happened. How could you be fine one minute and be screaming and pushing people out of the way the next? God, such a fool I made of myself. I must have looked a right mess cringing on the floor and crying my eyes out.

How could that doctor say I was fine? Did I forget to tell him about the dizziness and the pins and needles in my hands? God, what if he's missed a brain tumour?

It's a good job I stopped the train before it went into the tunnel. I'd have passed out for sure if the driver hadn't got me out in time. The heat in there! Thank God it wasn't a plane.

W**hat actually happened to Mary?** Her adrenaline levels reached red alert proportions and rocketed her into her first panic attack. Eventually, she put it down to the high levels of stress she'd been building up in the previous few days. She had flown into London to meet her boyfriend who was arriving on a long-haul flight from Sydney. She hadn't seen him for months and was looking forward to spending the weekend with him before they flew back home to Dublin together. She hadn't slept with excitement for the previous few nights. On top of that she'd been doing overtime to cover her costs.

That morning, on the way to meet his flight, Mary's taxi got gridlocked in rush hour traffic. She was going to be late! The driver, noticing how frantic she was, told her that she'd be quicker going by the underground from Victoria station. Dressed to kill, this was not what Mary wanted to hear. She'd planned this meeting for months and wanted to meet Larry looking great. They would run into each other's arms like it happens in the movies. But, taking the steps two at a time in a tight skirt and high heels, Mary felt her vision slipping away. She would never normally use the underground because she hated enclosed crowded places.

By the time she'd boarded the train she felt hot, sweaty and stressed-out. Breathless, she looked around for a seat, but there was standing room only. Her head began to swim. Her thoughts raced. *I'm going to be late, I'm not going to make it. Where's my mobile? God, I've left it in the hotel! Jesus it's hot in here, there's no air. . .*

T**he word 'panic' derives from Greek mythology.** Pan was the god of shepherds and flocks. He was depicted as half-man, half-animal, with a reed pipe, a shepherd's crook and a crown of pine leaves. He had horns, a wrinkled face and a very prominent chin. His body was hairy, the lower part of which was that of a male goat with cloven hoofs. He was adept at hiding, loving nothing better than his afternoon nap. He avenged himself on those who disturbed him with a sudden blood curdling screech, causing them to run for their lives.

The experience of a *panic* attack has parallels with this myth. Suddenly your body is in a state of emergency. You feel totally out of control, terrorised and in the grip of an irrational state of mind, with an overwhelming urge to flee to safety. This scenario is adrenaline-driven. You have been hijacked by one of your own molecules!

What distinguishes panic from anxiety, which is caused by a constant 'drip' of adrenaline, is that in panic the chemical is released in a *sudden dam-burst* which floods the body. Since adrenaline receptors are found in every cell in the body, the experience is widespread and affects every system: the cardiovascular, the respiratory, the gastrointestinal, the neurological and even the skin.

PORTRAIT OF PANIC

- **You feel light-headed**, dizzy, disoriented and on the point of fainting. You doubt if your jelly legs can support you as far as the nearest exit.
- **You may notice fleeting sensations of pins and needles** in your hands and numbness around your lips. Blurring or double vision makes it difficult to focus normally.
- **Trembling in your hands** can be so bad that you can't hold a cup or write a cheque.
- **There never seems to be enough air.** 'Where's the window' thoughts fill your mind. You take short panting breaths, or feel yourself choking or smothering. Every breath feels like it might be your last. 'Getting outside' is a question of survival.
- **Waves of hot and cold chills pass through you.** You want to take off layers and undo buttons. How you wish you could splash your face with cold water or plunge your hands into a bucket of ice-cubes! Your hands are clammy and sweat rolls off you. At night the sheets get saturated and need changing.

- **You are sure you are about to vomit**. Waves of nausea convince you that you are going to make a social spectacle of yourself. Crampy pains in your gut tell you to get to the bathroom now and allow the bout of diarrhoea to run its course.
- **A fast thumping heartbeat** terrifies you and you may believe that you are having a heart attack. Chest tightness and shooting pains down your arms confirm your worst fears. By this stage you may want to get the doctor or call the ambulance.
- **The pressure in your head** convinces you that you are about to burst a blood vessel in your brain. If this is not the first time it has happened, you might think you have a brain tumour.

THE AFTERMATH

Since a panic attack is such a terrifying life-and-death experience, it leaves a deep imprint. Many would say a death imprint. Like an earthquake, it is not easily forgotten or brushed aside. It dominates thinking and demands an explanation.

There is also an ominous feeling that something is seriously wrong. For this reason it is easy to see how individuals, in searching for an explanation, can believe that they may have had a heart attack, a stroke, are suffering from a yet undiagnosed brain tumour, have early multiple sclerosis or that they are going mad.

Spurred on by their fear, visits to the Accident and Emergency Departments are insisted upon. The family doctor is pressurised for answers and referrals may follow. Cardiology, neurology and respiratory departments are attended in search of a definitive diagnosis.

What makes panic attacks so mystifying for a sufferer is that they leave no physical trace. Like a train moving through a station, which creates a lot of noise and wind, the adrenaline leaves no evidence behind as its level rises and falls. Medical findings such as ECGs, X-rays, brain scans and blood tests are all negative. Paradoxically, this is not always good news! Nothing has yet explained the source of sufferers' intense and terrifying physical experiences, particularly if they have had more panic attacks in the meantime.

Many now become *pilgrim patients*, going from doctor to

doctor trying to put their mind at rest with a satisfactory explanation. Physical medicine by its very nature relates only to what
is visible and measurable, therefore if nothing can be found
then eventually everyone concludes that 'it's psychological'. This
may not sit easy with someone who, some days earlier, in the
throes of the panic attack was convinced they were dying! It is
inconceivable for them to believe — having survived 'certain
death' — that its source could be in the mind. 'What? My doctor wants me to take psychiatric drugs!'

Now reluctantly on medication and coping with side effects,
if panic continues to break through disillusionment sets in. Sufferers feel increasingly misunderstood, alienated and more
afraid than ever. Losing confidence in the medical profession,
they believe that something has been 'missed'. Onward goes our
pilgrim patient.

AWAKENING THE MONSTER

Having a panic attack is like waking up a ferocious beast.
Once aroused, it rips and roars through you, unstoppable
and out of control, terrifying you. When it departs, it leaves you
shocked, exhausted, disillusioned and beaten up.

In between attacks the monster sleeps and you tiptoe
around it. You are paranoid. You are on guard all the time. Who
wants another terrifying life-threatening experience? Your only
hope is to keep it from wakening, because once it is on the
move, you are dinner! You quickly learn that prevention is your
best policy and begin avoiding adrenaline-loaded triggers coming from both inside and out. Convinced that some mad thing
has taken up residence inside you, which in spite of your best
efforts is always trying to break out, you question your sanity.
'I'm cracking up, I'm going mad!'

BECOMING YOUR OWN BODYGUARD

Imagine your response if your home was broken into, not once,
not twice, but three or four times in the same week. After
these breaches of security, you would be thinking of little else.
Suspending your normal routines, battening down the hatches,
you would turn your house into a bunker. This is what life is
like if you are a panicker, all the worse because *the attack is*

from within. You are sleeping with the enemy. You live in constant dread because there is no place left to hide. All your thoughts, feelings and behaviours are focussed on preventing another attack — it is full catastrophe living.

This vigilance makes perfect sense, as such 'scanning' of the environment allows you to identify a threat in advance and get ready to escape. It is your radar system. 'How safe am I?' is all you think about. You'll even use it to check out your own body.

Physical activities raise your heart rate, make you sweat more and leave you breathless. Normally these changes aren't a problem. If you're a panicker, however, you may have learned to associate them with an imminent attack. If so, you'll avoid any activity that causes them. Heated arguments, watching exciting sports, sex, running upstairs and warm sweaty environments such as a bar or club, are tricky.

You become defensive and feel besieged. Inside and outside you are never off duty. The fight-flight response is never far away.

After a number of attacks you become acutely aware of situations that can trigger them off. For example, crowded places, long queues, or anywhere you cannot get out of quickly and simply. Many avoid the context in which the first panic attack occurred and consequently will not return to shopping malls, go on a plane, enter churches, cinemas, bars, clubs, hairdressers, etc. 'Avoidance of the marketplace' is the literal meaning of *agoraphobia*.

If avoidance is not possible, adaptive strategies are next. You can get there with the help of a drink en route, or as long as you have a tranquilliser on board. Life can continue as it was, once you always bring somebody else along, sit near exits, alter your working schedule to avoid heavy traffic, carry a mobile phone or eat on your own. Props such as a bike or a buggy, mean you do not have to worry about feeling dizzy and falling.

However, these manoeuvres make life complicated. It is difficult to explain to others why you have to leave the movie *now*, why you will not go shopping and cannot stand in a queue. Misunderstood, you may find yourself open to the ridicule and the intense irritation of others. Loathe to divulge your secret, you fob them off with excuses and cringe inwardly at their reaction.

A LIFE ON HOLD

With your eye always on the lookout for danger signals, your focus is forced to shift from the demands of everyday life to emergency mode. You are living in two parallel worlds, one competing with the other: the world of everyday routine versus the world of panic stations. If your attention cannot be in two places at once, there is no contest. Raw survival will always win. Lack of concentration, poor attention span and memory lapses now create extra stress. Balancing the two worlds consumes enormous amounts of energy, leaving you chronically irritable, frustrated and drained.

The thought of having a panic attack in front of others can be a fate worse than death. Many fear being misunderstood and judged harshly. 'They'll think I'm drunk, drugged, weird, strange or mad! The embarrassment!' Sufferers' thoughts run amok. What if you vomit in a restaurant, scream some obscenity in church or try to open the emergency exit door on a plane during take-off?

Next to the fear of making an absolute fool of yourself in public is the fear of being 'outed' as a panicker. It must be kept a secret at all costs. You might not even confide in your closest relatives and friends. The panicker's preoccupation with the judgement and criticism of others, *the public gaze*, feeds into the stigma associated with all mental distress. This paranoia leads to loneliness and alienation.

Self-loathing and shame are inevitable travelling companions of this crippling condition. 'I'm so stupid to be reacting like this, I'm useless, I'd be better off dead'. These are depressing thoughts and panic masks many a diagnosis of depression.

LET'S ASK OUR PANEL OF EXPERTS

Professor Moore (mind-brain specialist): 'Panic is such an all-or-nothing condition. One minute you're standing calmly in a queue and the next you're charging for the door. This is so because panic acts as a survival reflex. It's automatic and involuntary. It's a primitive protective response, set in motion when a threat is perceived by the limbic or reptilian part of our brain. That's our "old brain" and being protective, it overrides the voluntary rational "new brain". That's the grey matter that forms our neocortex.

'Reflexes act instantly and involuntarily. If you trip, your arms automatically shoot out in front of you to break your fall. If your cortex had to be consulted, the process would be so slow that you'd have fallen on your face before the answer came. This explains why a panicker's behaviours may seem out of control, nonsensical and stupid to others. They say things like: "Before I knew where I was, I found myself running out of the supermarket" or "If I didn't get off that plane I would have lost my mind." They feel utterly taken over and hijacked by their own basic survival instinct. Panic is the "flight" part of the fight-flight response. Just like Mary on the train, "I'm outta here." '

Joe (layperson): 'I can understand Mary's panic on the train, travelling makes lots of people tense. Running out of a place she goes to every day, one that's she's obviously so familiar with, does not make sense. What could have caused today's panic attack?'

Professor Moore (mind-brain specialist): 'Panic is about life and death. She thought she was going to suffocate on the train and ever since then she associates warm crowded places with that memory. The very thought of standing in a queue in public makes her adrenaline levels go through the roof — that speeds up her breathing, her heart starts racing and she thinks she's going to lose control. By avoiding coming in here she protects herself from the danger of that feeling happening again. So technically she has developed a *phobia*, a conditioned response, which makes perfect sense. It reduces risk.'

Ruth (psychotherapist): 'People get phobias about all sorts of things. It's their way of dealing with fear and the feeling of being out of control. If they can project their fear outside themselves by putting it on something concrete which they can avoid, then they feel more in control and safer. "If I don't go near the supermarket, I'll be fine."

'Mary, like many others, has associated her fear of the suffocating sensations with certain places only. This gives them a measure of control, otherwise they'd never be able to relax. Most feel safest at home.

'I see a lot of stressed-out business people who get panic attacks. Typically they're burnt-out, overloaded with work, not sleeping and working to tight deadlines. Their concentration and memory have begun to let them down. I had an executive recently who had to flee the boardroom during a tense meeting. Normally a competent man, he'd made a few errors of judgement lately which were on his mind. It was at the end of a busy day and he was already awash with adrenaline. When he was asked a simple question, he went blank in mid-sentence, got into a terrible state and had to excuse himself. He was taken totally by surprise. This was so "not" him.

'Many like him have a Type A personality. They're the ones who drive themselves too hard and don't know when to stop. Delegation doesn't come easily to them and they're always in competition with the clock. He'll have to learn to say "no" more often, manage his boundaries and have more realistic expectations of himself in order to reduce his adrenaline and prevent future attacks.

'It's essential that anyone having panic attacks or suffering from high anxiety should go for relaxation training, where they'll learn to control the symptoms during an attack and to prevent them. If they learn diaphragmatic or abdominal breathing, the feelings of suffocation and symptoms such as dizziness can be controlled. Biofeedback helps them learn this more quickly through the use of computerised technology which measures such variables as muscle tension, sweat response, hand temperature and heart rate. They can see on screen the effect their adrenaline is having on their bodies. Also they can see how these can be altered and normalised by the combination of abdominal breathing, peaceful thoughts and visualisations. Seeing is believing.

'With such skills in place they start to feel safer and safer and have fewer fear thoughts which then disappear altogether. Once these thoughts are out of the way, their effects, the high levels of adrenaline which generate the panic attacks, stop.'

Jackie (energy therapist): 'There's another aspect to panic. It's about social identity, role and what people think of us. The issue of the public gaze has an enormous impact on all our lives. We can become preoccupied with being the "right" kind of person and expend huge amounts of energy to that end. It is through this created identity that we come to know ourselves and we prefer if it stays the same. This familiarity makes us feel secure. You know yourself to be: honest, loyal, a team player, an excellent home-maker, a good parent, an adequate provider, physically attractive, mentally strong, competent, reliable etc.

'If you find yourself in a situation where any part of that identity is now in doubt where, for example, you've been called a liar, or accused of not pulling your weight, you will naturally feel undermined. This sends danger signals through your system and is interpreted as a threat to your very existence — your social existence. It's a form of social death. If you can't protect this image of yourself through circumstances outside your control, you'll start to panic.

'This is why people may begin having panic attacks when their marriage ends, following unemployment, redundancy or disability, if they fail an exam, if they don't get the expected promotion, if they develop a sexual dysfunction, if a misdemeanor has been discovered or they're wrongly accused of something.

Losing "face" is the issue here — I call it Public Gaze Panic.

'The chakra system (see Appendix) is identity-oriented and provides a scaffolding for the personality. Consequently anything that threatens to annihilate our core identity puts the chakra system, in particular the third chakra, into chaos. "How do I handle this?"

'Energetically the focus of a panic attack is on the third chakra. That's the one which normally deals with personal power, will, individuality and which gives us the ability to influence our lives. The verb of the third is "I can". "I can take care of myself, handle things, protect myself and control my life." It's the very opposite of panic, in which there is no leader, no manager.

'With the personality in doubt and without leadership, the energy is dissipated in many directions throughout the chakra system. This explains the totality of the experience, which affects every cell and every system in the body. The energetic response to this chaos is to simplify matters and boil it all down to life and death. The first chakra gets charged and starts making survival decisions on behalf of the entire system. This is why panickers will do things in certain situations as though their life depended on it.'

Patrick (spiritual healer): 'If ever the issue of our own mortality arises it reverberates throughout the system, pressing all the buttons. It's a red alert! Death anxiety often comes up after major surgery, following a bereavement, after the diagnosis of a life-threatening illness or surviving a near-fatal road traffic accident. Anything with the theme of death can be terrifying.

'Given that death is an inevitability, it's surprising how little attention we give to it. More often than not we try to sweep it under the carpet and put off the day when we can no longer avoid addressing it. We try our best to keep it outside of awareness, buried safely away in our unconscious mind.

'We've all heard the stories of people who may have walked away from a serious road traffic accident, bounced back from bypass surgery or supported a loved one through a life-threatening illness — then out of the blue, months later, just when things had returned to normal they found themselves experiencing panic attacks. Their existential fear of death has suddenly surfaced.

'Fears about death take different forms. Some are about the afterlife, some are about the actual process of dying. Some even fear being buried alive! For others there's the fear of not having the time to realize their full potential, or of leaving their family and loved ones bereft. Whatever way it's fertile ground for panic.

'This is where psychotherapy is so important. It can help sufferers to make the link between an experience where they could have died and their present-day panic attack, so they understand that the two events are connected — then their panic attack makes sense and isn't so "out of the blue" after all.

'Another thing that makes panic attacks so unexpected is that in our culture panic never gets talked about — it's a well-kept secret. As a result children never hear about it and if they themselves ever get a panic attack, they don't know what's happening to them or what to do about it. Consequently, as is the case with all unfamiliar phenomena, they fear it. Look at what happens in childbirth. A lot of mothers are out of their minds with fear. Their labour pains aren't all they're screaming about!

'Panic is a dramatic reminder of the fragility of the physical body. Just how impermanent life is and how caught up we can become in our beliefs and attachments, even to life. As with all serious symptoms, panic attacks are a wake-up call to our spiritual dimension and the need for soul-attending.

'Karmically, panic presents us with a predicament which we can learn from — how to deal with the uncertainty and unpredictability of the earth plane, as well as learning not to be so attached to certainty and our past conditioning. It challenges us to let go of our fear of death, so that we can free up the energy of creation — the life-force. If our energy becomes tied up in shielding us from our fear of death, it's not available for the purpose of living life to its full spiritual potential.

'The same is true of the public gaze. Vast amounts of energy are haemorrhaged into maintaining a social façade. Many become slaves to their social identity, their carefully constructed role and wouldn't have a self if that disappeared. This state flies in the face of our very reason for being here, namely to discover who we are as individuals. First know thyself.'

Dr Clarke (homeopath): 'Working with the life-force has become central to the way I work. I sense its presence in everything and observe it in its most evolved form in a human being. When I prescribe a remedy it's for the purpose of removing whatever may be standing in the way of its full expression. I see a remedy as analogous to a tuning fork, harmonising the wavelengths of the body's electromagnetic energy field. When the body is in tune or in perfect balance, the life-force can express itself most powerfully. Health is not just about the absence of disease.

'It's my view that states of imbalance in a homeopathic sense correlate with energetic imbalance as reflected in the chakras and energy field. No-one to my knowledge has linked these two disciplines in terms of energetic effect. References to chakras are not to be found in homeopathic texts. Since both homeopathy and bioenergy heal by vibrational means it seems inevitable that a conversation will open up between the two of them in the future.

'Look at panic as a case in point. Many of the remedies that I would use target the first and third chakra issues. **Aconite** is indicated when panic is secondary to an overwhelming fear of death. I prescribe **Kali Arsenicum** when there is a tremendous anxiety about health, particularly when a heart attack is perceived as imminent. **Argentum Nitricum** is one of the principle remedies for anticipatory anxiety, the feeling that something awful will happen or that they will do something impulsive. This is the public gaze type of panic and is good for claustrophobia and agoraphobia. Mary would benefit from this remedy. **Phosphorus** eases the anxiety that comes with having poor boundaries, for those who are easily overstimulated by their environment, becoming inundated and exhausted by the demands of outside world.'

Dr Henry (psychiatrist): 'Because of my medical training I see psychological distress as a disease — as pathology, as a condition to be diagnosed and treated with the appropriate medication. I see panic attacks as reflecting an underlying chemical imbalance with a genetic component. Newer psychoactive medications are being developed all the time, thanks to the substantial investments by pharmaceutical companies into the area of research and drug trials. It is only a question of time before panic disorders will be effectively controlled and eradicated.'

CHAPTER 10 — POST-TRAUMATIC STRESS DISORDER

Keynote: The Alarm That Won't Stop

Isabel **was sexually assaulted** in her home five years ago. She had two young children aged three and eleven months. A new carpet was due to be delivered and fitted. When the doorbell rang she was confronted with a man pulling a balaclava over his face. He forced his way inside and attacked her wielding a knife. He threatened to kill the children if she didn't do what he asked. Ordering her upstairs he locked the children in the bathroom and dragged Isabel into the bedroom. He beat her, tore some of her clothes off and knocked her to the ground, attempting to rape her. The more she resisted the more violent he became.

Isabel remembers drifting in and out of consciousness several times, hearing the children screaming. On one occasion she was convinced she was going to die. She found herself looking down on her body from above, being slashed with a knife. A voice said, 'Go back, they need you.' With that she returned to her body and naked and bleeding, found herself racing down the stairs and running out onto the street. The rapist escaped through the back door.

In the aftermath, Isabel could not get the images out of her mind. All she could see was the rapist's eyes, the knife and blood everywhere. She kept hearing his voice repeating, 'Shut your mouth bitch, if you don't stop screaming I'll kill ya.' So overwhelming were the images that Isabel often felt that she was reliving the attack. These flashbacks left her terrified and led to horrific panic attacks, often causing her to run to a neighbour's house seeking help. When these became a daily occurrence, her husband took time off work.

Nightly she would wake screaming, suffocating and soaked in sweat. She needed endless reassurance that the attack was over and that he was not coming back. In the months that followed Isabel's life changed radically. She lost her confidence, became socially withdrawn, depressed and mistrustful. She avoided sex and became increasingly clingy and dependent on her husband. Her only security was knowing that he was contactable by mobile phone at all times. If she could not reach him a panic attack would instantly follow. She would flee the house with the children even if they'd been asleep and drive frantically to his workplace.

There were no longer any mirrors in the house, because when Isabel looked into one she would see blood-spattered walls behind her. She would only sleep or have a bath if her husband was home, fearing the attacker would return. Her fear and paranoia were such that the family eventually moved to a new house. Isabel's moods ranged from passivity to sudden rage. She would frequently smash things, while at other times she would weep for hours. Her memory often let her down and her attention span was so short that she could no longer read, previously her main hobby. Despite medication and immersion in various counselling programmes, little changed in Isabel's life. Her out-of-body experience frightened her — it raised questions about death which she found disturbing. She kept obsessively playing over in her mind how life had been before the attack. Unable to let it go, the question 'Why me?' haunted her. She blamed herself for not checking before she opened the door to the attacker.

Post-traumatic stress disorder (PTSD) may develop if you witness or experience a traumatic event involving actual or threatened death or bodily harm and to which your response is intense fear, helplessness or horror. Road traffic accidents, plane crashes, violent assaults, rape, natural disasters and war etc. are all common sources of PTSD. Life-threatening events can leave a *death imprint*.

PTSD can also result from feelings of helplessness and utter lack of control in the face of wilful traumas such as torture and sexual abuse which relates to a death of another kind — *soul death*. Fear of death is instinctive. Every living organism has an in-built avoidance reflex which is triggered by life-threatening situations. It is a *protective survival response* whose job is to keep us alive and safe from harm.

Taken Over by the Reptilian Persona

In the core of the human brain is the ancient limbic or 'reptilian' nervous tissue. It is millions of years old and is still a major player. When it needs to, it has the power to override the programmes of the newer parts of the brain, principally the neocortex, the seat of rational, logical thought and self-awareness.

When we are confronted with a life-threatening situation this reptile part instantaneously propels us, using the innate emotions of rage and fear, into the fight-flight response. This emergency response is automatic and involuntary — a reflex. It is *independent of will* and once instinctively turned on, it cannot be turned off by will alone.

Once the trauma is over, this part of the brain shifts its focus to the future in order to make us more aware of danger, sharpen our survival reactions and in so doing prevent a possible recurrence. It does this by repeatedly rerunning the traumatic event in our mind and in our dreams, like a security video it attempts to scan every detail. It is looking for any possible slip-up in your attention which may have initially exposed you to the trauma. The 'video' will continue running in your mind night and day, also reminding you of the feelings you experienced at the time. These emotionally charged images will not stop until your reptile brain is satisfied that the 'higher levels' have 'got the message' and that safety measures have been put in place.

Portrait of PTSD

- **Hypervigilant**, your adrenaline running high, you are on guard and wary all the time. Suspicious and paranoid you blow things out of proportion. Panic is never far away. You often feel your heart racing, your breathing laboured and you sweat profusely. Your muscles can go into tension spasms — tremors are common.
- **You startle easily**, jumping in alarm to a sudden sound such as a door banging or the phone ringing.
- **One of the first casualties is sleep**, which is also one of the last things to return to normal. This causes extreme fatigue and allows no let-up from the constant barrage of mental imagery. Your mind is in 'on mode' all the time.
- **Intrusive vivid images** of the event haunt you, replaying the trauma over and over without mercy. Such is their intensity that you feel as if you have been catapulted back into the initial trauma as if re-experiencing it for the first time. These flashbacks can occur when least expected. Jim, who survived a road traffic accident, would find himself at his desk or at the family dinner table clinging to an imaginary steering wheel, urgently honking the

horn and shouting 'Get back on your own side, get back on your own side!' His mind was literally reliving the head-on collision in which his girlfriend was killed.

- **This persistent re-running of traumatic events** on your screen of perception is comparable to a Vietnam vet, newly returned from the front, being repeatedly compelled to watch the horrific opening scenes of the war movie *Saving Private Ryan*. Every re-run reopens the original trauma and what is so frightening and despairing about them is that they cannot be voluntarily stopped. You get frustrated trying to explain to others how something in the past could still be so 'real' in the present. Months later smells, sounds and tactile sensations may remain vivid and disturbing. Three years on Steve, a policeman serving with a rapid response unit, could still smell the gunpowder of a Kalashnikov rifle which was discharged at him at close range.

- **Nightmares destroy your sleep** and can be so terrifying that you eventually dread the moment when you close your eyes. You regularly wake soaked in sweat and in the middle of a panic attack. Bizarre sleep patterns become the norm and sleep deprivation is common.

- **Avoidance strategies**. In a desperate effort to control your escalating anxiety levels you avoid everything associated with the event. You try not to talk about it and you avoid the scene of the trauma or any reminders of it, such as TV programmes. If you have survived a car crash you will postpone driving. If you have been raped, having sex can trigger a flashback.

- **Emotionally you are on a roller coaster.** You experience the full spectrum — panic, anger and rage, episodes of crying and sadness. Feelings of hopelessness and despair become the norm. As a result, being in the company of others becomes an extra stress because of the unpredictable and trigger-hair nature of your emotional outbursts. Ordinary life is merely a memory. Suicide passes through your mind — 'I don't want to be here.'

- **Paranormal experiences** that occurred at the time of the traumatic event are difficult to make sense of and therefore your mind is drawn to them. Such experiences include time standing still (where the traumatic events happen in slow motion), apparitions and visions of dead loved ones, 'out of body' and 'near death' experiences.

From a viewpoint outside your body you may have felt
that you were looking down on yourself while trapped
in a car, on the operating table, or in the process of
being attacked. It's as though you were watching a
drama unfolding in which you were the main player.
While being raped at knifepoint in the back of a car,
Jean remembers looking down on herself and at the
same time being comforted by her dead grandmother,
who held her in her arms, whispering over and over,
'You'll be OK, you'll be OK.'

- **The 'near death' experience** has the added distinction of
  the sensation of moving up a tunnel, at the end of which
  is a white light, perceived as being the next life. There,
  you may have met dead relatives or heard a voice from
  the earth plane calling you back. While being wheeled
  into an operating theatre with multiple injuries, David
  felt that he was dying. He experienced himself travelling
  up a tunnel and emerging into a light-filled area. It was
  like a 'football stadium full of spirits' with his dead relatives standing at the entrance. He was deeply upset that
  his mother, to whom he had been so close, instead of
  welcoming him said, 'Go back, your time hasn't come.'

- **Shutdown and shock**. It can seem as though you are
  looking at life from behind a glass pane. A state of emergency reigns. You may feel totally dislodged or fractured
  from your usual ways of thinking, feeling and behaving.
  'Normality' has disappeared. You feel alienated, split off,
  de-skilled, dazed and anxious. You wonder if you are
  mad. Your work, leisure and family life is turned upside
  down.

- **You live in parallel universes** — your ordinary life and
  your extra-ordinary inner world. Because you are in
  emergency mode, you can focus on nothing else but the
  trauma and what will become of you. As a result of not
  being fully present, you have trouble with your short-
  term memory, your attention span is limited and poor
  concentration is the norm. Inevitably you make mistakes
  and lose confidence in your ability to carry out simple
  tasks. You start to feel 'stupid' as names are forgotten,
  car keys are lost, conversations become difficult to follow and the execution of routine tasks requires more
  focus which exceeds your capabilities. Your inner movie
  constantly distracts you.

- **Emotional numbing**. You may find that after six months or more, in an effort to dampen down your emotional distress, you unconsciously anaesthetise your feelings — you 'numb out'. Feeling as if you are in limbo, much like the 'walking dead', you merely go through the motions of living. You neither express emotion nor register the feelings of others. This state of suspended animation can be extremely distressing for those around you, making them angry and concerned as you become ever more unreachable. 'He's in his own world and has tuned out what's going on around him. A train could pass through the house and he wouldn't notice!'

- **Collateral damage**. Another way of numbing your pain and inducing sleep is to use alcohol and other substances. As you increasingly withdraw into your own world, your relationships suffer, deadlines cease to exist and problems at work arise. Now chronically awash with adrenaline, suspicion and paranoia increasingly alienate you from others. In order to distract yourself, to the annoyance of others, you keep frantically busy and 'on the run' from the feelings and images which flood in as soon as you stop. Out of character behaviours such as gambling and promiscuity can begin. Feeling you have nothing to lose, you might engage in reckless behaviours and expose yourself to unnecessary risks. The character played by Jeff Bridges who survived an air disaster in the film *Fearless* is a good example of a PTSD sufferer. He balanced on the ledge of a tall building, jaywalked through fast-flowing traffic, drove his car into a wall and ate food to which he was known to be dangerously allergic.

- **You feel misunderstood by others**. Much to your surprise, sympathy and support for your difficulties is time-limited and starts to wane. A recognised ritual exists in traumas such as bereavement, whereby support is given immediately and recognition of the impact acknowledged. Flowers, cards, phone calls and practical help follow. There are no similar rituals in place for the post-traumatised individual, who can feel ignored and rejected. After a number of weeks questions may be asked of you, like 'When will things settle back to normal?' and 'Shouldn't you be back in the saddle by now?' Subtle innuendoes are made which have a judgemental air about them. 'He

looks fine and he's able to mow the lawn, why isn't he
back at work?' It may be inferred that you are 'playing it
up', 'malingering', or 'milking the system'.

- **Socially you withdraw**, fearing the judgement of others.
  Now it's easier to avoid situations where you might have
  to explain yourself. Doors are not answered, phone calls
  are not taken and you start living like a recluse. Bitterness and cynicism may set in. If you had your way you
  would hide away in some isolated sanctuary. There you
  would be free to eat and sleep when you wanted, act
  out your distress without concerning others and have no
  responsibilities.

- **Past the heal-by date**. As the months and years roll by,
  you are shocked that normality has not returned yet.
  'How can it take so long?' You become increasingly frustrated and impatient with the healing time-frame. A beautiful insight into this was unfolded in the book and film
  The Horse Whisperer, the story of a post-traumatically
  stressed horse named Pilgrim, who was brought to a
  horse whisperer for healing. The owners of the horse, on
  pressing the horse-whisperer for a definitive heal-by date
  were always greeted with his knowing reply: 'That
  depends on Pilgrim.' He acknowledged the unique
  nature of the horse and its healing time-frame, which
  could only be assisted but not hurried. Impatience had
  no place here.

- **Grief eclipsed**. Your anxiety can be so much in the fore-
  ground and your mind in such turmoil, that there is often
  no room for grieving for what has been lost. This could
  be the loss of a physical function through disability,
  loved ones who died in the same trauma, or your career
  and financial earning power. You may sense a dam-burst
  of grief awaiting when the mental spin-cycle stops.

- **The problem of the 'extra piece'**. Before long you know
  you'll never be the same again. You are like Humpty
  Dumpty falling off the wall, breaking into hundreds of
  pieces. On attempting to rebuild yourself you find extra
  pieces, which means that your life cannot be rebuilt in
  exactly the same way again. The pieces of the traumatic experience are just too different to be incorporated.
  Where before you may have fitted hand in glove into a
  couple relationship or a working life, now you may feel
  at odds, sensing that there is a mismatch.

- **Fear of stigma**. You may be the kind of person who has always been wary of psychoactive medication and the last place you ever imagined ending up in was a psychiatric hospital. Suggestions that you need one or the other can be terrifying, confirming your worst fears that you are going mad.

PTSD: Wilful and Perceptual Trauma

It would be a mistake to think that PTSD only results from your own possible death, accidental or otherwise. You may have witnessed a traumatic event second-hand, such as happens if you work in any of the emergency services, as medics, ambulance crew, police etc. Likewise those coming to terms with the horrific injuries of a loved one can suffer from PTSD-by-proxy. Carol is a case in point. Watching TV at home, Carol got a phone call informing her that her husband and two daughters were involved in a road traffic accident. On arriving at the hospital she was unprepared for the news. Her youngest daughter was dead on arrival, while the other daughter and husband were in operating theatres fighting for their lives. He did not survive and her daughter suffered permanent brain damage.

Some other traumas have an extra layer to them. These are the ones where the trauma involved a wilful, premeditated act with a deeply personal aspect to it. In other words, *I was chosen and not someone else*, to be bullied, threatened, sexually abused or raped. Now we are inevitably forced to ask ourselves the question, 'What was it about me that caused me to be singled out?' Our radar system needs to know, in the interest of future prevention. 'Did I do anything to bring it on myself?' We become plagued with guilt and shame, which is made all the worse by the intimate nature of the trauma and the fact that guilt and shame are less easily put into words and shared than the physical details of an event such as an accident.

What is also deeply disturbing to us about these traumas is the profound questions they raise about human nature. The mind seeks to know, 'Why would somebody want to inflict so much pain on me or anybody else? What kind of monster would commit such acts?' The very essence of humanity comes under review. How does a child make sense of their father, uncle or neighbour sexually abusing them? How does a twelve-year-old face his peers who spit at him and call him 'gay'? How does a single mum cope with the dilemma of needing the job to support herself and two children, while fending off the predatorial sexual advances of her boss? These are not idle rhetorical questions, they are once again part of our intelligent radar system, hoping to identify and prevent similar threats in the future.

Many therapists working with the survivors of sexual abuse, rape or torture, describe how their clients feel as if they have been robbed, not just of their innocence, but of some inner light, leaving them lifeless. It is as if their very *soul has been eclipsed*. If the trauma is not fully processed in therapy at an early stage, it may present itself many years later as self-mutilation, suicidal behaviour, bulimia, anorexia, obsessive-compulsive disorders, substance misuse, sexual disorientation or dysfunctional relationships. The painful process of peeling back the layers within a psychotherapeutic relationship so that they can be verbalised and integrated is a lengthy one, sometimes without any satisfactory resolution, so all-pervasive is this soul damage.

In a consumer society we often feel that our status and quality of life reflects on our inner worth. As a result, many people are becoming victims of the public gaze. Our point of reference as to how 'good' a person we are is measured by the trappings of success. We live through our role and the status it provides. Unfortunately our inner or true self becomes obscured by how we 'should be', or 'have to be' in order to get approval. With no internal reference point and less and less spiritual awareness, there is often no inner self to fall back on when trauma occurs. A marriage breaking down, being passed over for promotions or the loss of a job can be as traumatic for some as a death! It is a *social death*. When our public identity changes and we are seen in all our vulnerability — subject to the judgement of others — metaphorically we can feel annihilated. It is a *perceptual* trauma. Our reason for living has been ripped from under our feet. Many commit suicide because of such social deaths.

PTSD with a Lost 'T': The Unintegrated Experience

Some distressed individuals have all the signs of PTSD, with one exceptional feature. They have *no conscious memory* of having had a traumatic event happen to them. Although they may be having daily panic attacks, horrific nightmares, hyper-vigilance etc, the cause is a source of mystery.

Frequently, early childhood traumas of a physical or sexual nature remain unhealed. The trauma was never recognised and never treated. At the time of the abuse these children were not developmentally equipped to handle the intensity of such experiences, or to put it into words. Their inability to process the trauma at the time meant that it became *sealed off in their unconscious mind and as such obscured from their awareness.* It is nonetheless stored within their energy field and chakra system (see Appendix) where it is constantly expressed as an imbalance. In this form it travels with them through the rest of their childhood into adult life. Many carry it to the grave.

Tragically along this time line, although beyond awareness, PTSD is still very much alive in terms of its effects. In childhood these include acting-out behaviours, learning disabilities, bed-wetting, dysfluency, truancy, delinquency and other maladjusted behaviours. In adult life they may be expressed as psychosomatic disorders, sexual dysfunction, depression, eating disorders, substance abuse, obsessive-compulsive disorders, psychosis, self-mutilation, suicidal behaviours, personality disorders, acts of violence and other serious crimes.

Imagine having daily images of faces suddenly bearing down on top of you, flashbacks of body parts covered in blood, accompanied by the kinaesthetic feelings of stubble against your cheek and the smell of alcohol or sperm? Imagine if the only way to prevent a terrifying panic attack is to lock your bedroom door every night, wear protective layers of clothes in bed and avoid intimacy of any kind — and you do not even know the reason why. Ultimately you will take the view that you are weird and feel that you are on the road to madness. Over the years you'll come to loathe and despise yourself for these peculiarities, holding yourself responsible. Why wouldn't you? There does not seem to be anybody else to blame. 'It must be me, I have a sick mind.'

I've come to realise that sexual assault is an imposed death experience for the victim. That is, the victim experiences her life as having been taken by someone else.   Evangeline Kane

LET'S ASK OUR PANEL OF EXPERTS

Joe (layperson): 'I can understand how people like Isabel and children who are sexually abused might never recover, but what about people who've been involved in horrific accidents? Some just seem to take it in their stride and get on with their lives.'

Ruth (psychotherapist): 'Research shows that there's no link between the pre-accident personality and PTSD. In other words, there's no way to predict how anyone would react when they look death in the face. There are thousands of variables in the pot, change any one of them and it makes the difference between business as usual and chaos for years. There seems to be no guarantee that PTSD will not happen to you after a trauma. I could be involved in an accident tonight and maybe in a few months time I will be struggling with PTSD!

'One thing that we think helps decrease the likelihood of that happening, however, is debriefing or crisis intervention. That's why they fly experts to the site of any major incident, such as a plane or train crash, to meet with the survivors and their relatives — it applies equally well to a rape or after a fire in the home. Even with the best of interventions the symptoms can last for years or a life-time. PTSD is a real rag-bag with every known symptom in it. In the end, getting over things is an extremely personal thing as it calls on survival resources which you may or may not have.

'One thing we're all seeing a lot more of these days is young people recovering from drug-induced trauma, who afterwards begin experiencing mental symptoms which terrify them. The overwhelming nature of these symptoms leave some people believing that they've caused permanent brain damage. This is particularly so if they're the only one of their group who has had such an experience. 'My brain is wrecked, I'll never be the same again.' Flashbacks, panic attacks, mood swings, insomnia and difficulty concentrating reinforce to them the belief that this is so. It can take months for them to settle. A minority go on to develop a schizophrenic-type state as a result of having been frightened by the feeling of their personal boundaries melting away, an effect induced by the 'oneness' experience of the drug, as well as being afraid they would be unable to re-establish them.'

Professor Moore (mind-brain specialist): 'That's understandable, since under the influence of the drug they feel they can't define themselves in the usual way. In this 'oceanic' experience, with their boundary gone, they have disappeared, they can't find themselves, metaphorically they've died!

'This trauma aside, once the death imprint has been registered by the brain for any reason, the primitive or limbic part moves to centre stage and expresses itself in its full terrifying ferocity. Sleep deprivation is a huge problem and the chemistry of the dreaming state can break through when sufferers are awake. It's like having a nightmare with your eyes wide open — a daymare! Terrifying stuff when your ordinary life is going on around you at the same time. A state of madness if ever there was one! To make matters worse you're running higher levels of adrenaline than you've ever run before. Many live in a state of perpetual panic.

'It is a common misconception that if you have enough willpower you can turn off the reptile which is playing havoc within you. The chemistry is extremely complex, as it involves our three brains; the reptilian, the mammalian and the neocortex. It's as if it was 'agreed' among them, that in life-threatening situations the primitive brain will be given executive rights over the others, in the interest of raw survival.

'The notion of expecting the neocortex to produce the chemistry of calm, by instructions such as 'Pull yourself together' in the middle of a survival crisis and its immediate aftermath, is ridiculous. The reptile brain doesn't respect our hopes and wishes, or indeed the advice or admonishments of others — its only interest is safety.

'Victims often chastise themselves after a rape for not 'putting up a fight'. They couldn't because their survival response, assessing the overall situation, decided chemically in favour of 'freeze' as the most life-supporting option — like the rabbit caught in the headlights of the car. They don't understand that it has nothing whatsoever to do with will or determination. Nobody should blame themselves for 'doing' this as it isn't a question of conscious choice.'

Ruth (psychotherapist): 'Many live with the guilt and shame for years. Psychotherapy is essential to help them to see that they did their very best at the time and deserve no blame or judgement. Paradoxically, the fact that women didn't 'struggle' during a rape used to be held against them in court. Young soldiers were executed as traitors and cowards in the trenches by their own side for showing signs of their own survival response, by refusing to go over the top or by running away. Later it became known as 'shell shock'.

'What a relief that nowadays we have the label PTSD for such a bewildering constellation of symptoms. This is particularly important for those who have been sexually abused as children and have never been able to make sense of what was wrong with them for so many years. It can be a very healing piece of information.'

Jackie (energy therapist): 'I see 'out-of-body' and 'near-death' experiences happening along a spectrum. It's a question of degree. They occur when the body's energy field gets prematurely separated from it, dislodged by the intensity of the trauma. What normally occurs in death is that the energy field gradually separates from the body and finally leaves it only after it's already dead. Explanations like these are crucial to those who feel that these strange experiences must indicate that they are teetering on the edge of madness. In this way they're demystified and normalised.

'In PTSD the chakra system is thrown into imbalance and there are disturbances within and between the layers of the energy field. Disruption and interference has occurred to their electromagnetic frequencies affecting the entire mind-body-spirit organism. Although there may be no evidence of physical injury, the emotional, mental and spiritual layers are absorbing the impact — they act like shock absorbers. It's cause and effect in action.

'Can you imagine the disturbed violent energy that your field would absorb if you were being raped? That's why victims feel so contaminated and continue to experience kinaesthetic sensations of, say, a hand in their vagina or the smell of sweat for years afterwards — feeling the very presence of the rapist. He actually is present — in the sufferer's energy field! Small wonder they feel disturbed. It is critical to understand this phenomenon as it makes sense of why victims are not able to get on with their lives and remain locked into the traumatic event. Energy workers and homeopaths understand this phenomenon.

'Because the energy field is in a state of shock and the energetic flow through the chakras is imbalanced and diminished, many of the human qualities of "being alive" are absent. They feel as if a glass pane separates them from the world around them. Many feel numb, detached and are like ghostly onlookers unable to engage or participate in their usual life. 'Life is passing me by.' With each chakra compromised, the area of life that it covers suffers. As a result the identifiable symptoms of energetic shutdown emerge.

'With an imbalanced first chakra there is a loss of drive and motivation. Sufferers lose interest in life because they don't have the energy to engage it. They feel tired all the time as well as drained. Everything is an effort, they're running on empty. 'I don't want to be here' is dominant. They can suffer from haemorrhoids, musculo-skeletal problems and immune deficiencies.

'At the second chakra their ability to experience pleasure and fun diminishes, they can't connect socially with people and avoid group activities, efforts to cheer them up fail. Alienation of friends and family is commonplace. Emotionally numb or blunted, they're disinterested in intimacy. Libido plummets, erectile dysfunction and irritable bowel are common.

'In their solar plexus (the centre of personal power) where their third chakra is located, there is an ever-decreasing sense of control, willpower and autonomy. They are 'not in the driving seat'. Their sense of helplessness is reinforced by the fact that they can't even control their own body. These individuals, who may have been competently running businesses and homes, are now frustrated to find they're unable to influence symptoms such as palpitations, panic attacks and episodes of weeping. Physically they may suffer from peptic ulcers.

'At the fourth chakra compassion and acceptance are difficult to access. As a result sufferers withdraw love from themselves and can't receive it from others. They feel mortally wounded, betrayed by life, hurt and abandoned. Many begin to experience chest tightness, hypertension and respiratory difficulties.

'Compromised at their fifth chakra they feel misunderstood and unable to express themselves adequately to others. They find it difficult to put into words how they are feeling and what they need. Isolation sets in and innovation and creativity dry up. The muscles of their neck and shoulders are stiff and painful.

'Clarity eludes people with no sixth chakra energy and they feel they've 'lost the plot'. They are plagued by poor memory, lapses in concentration and an inability to focus. Visualising a future is impossible. The negative energy of dis-illusionment, depression and despair permeates every cell in their body. At a physical level many experience sore eyes, blurred vision and frontal headaches.

'Since the seventh chakra relates to the spiritual dimension, when it becomes compromised many turn their back on religious beliefs and practices, becoming cynical. Questions such as 'What have I done to deserve this?' and 'Why me?' preoccupy them. Life becomes meaningless.'

Dr Clarke (homeopath): 'I had a patient recently who was held up at gunpoint when she interrupted a robbery in progress at her home. The intruder, believing there was a safe in the house, threatened to kill her if she didn't reveal its whereabouts.

When she finally convinced him that there was no safe, he bound and gagged her. Two hours later she was freed by her husband. Such was her distress that he brought her to the nearest Accident and Emergency Department. Soon after she developed appalling skin rashes and had an epileptic seizure. She did the rounds of doctors and was referred to me through a friend a year later.

'Angry red skin usually implies bottled-up explosive energy, but this certainly didn't describe my client who was always, even now, a quiet accepting person. I felt her symptoms were reflecting the impression left as an energy complex in her electromagnetic field by the violence of her assailant. I treated her with **Stramonium** and her rash rapidly disappeared. This is a homeopathic remedy which reflects the violent constitutional nature of some individuals. In prison populations it would be the predominant one found.

'Homeopathy is based on the principle of treating 'like with like'. In this way the robber's violent energy was released from my patient's energy field. Stramonium is also frequently used in children who've been abused — and for night terrors. Isabel was also violated and assaulted, so this remedy would be good for her. In the early stages following many violent traumas it's better to give **Aconite** for the associated death anxiety and panic. In fact Aconite can be used to release a shock or fright that's been held in the body or mind for a lifetime.

'When the body has been injured, hurt or shocked more than the mind, **Arnica** becomes the remedy to help the individual release and heal the trauma. The Arnica state is characterised by an internal fragility that is threatened by just the approach or touch of another person. Chronic states of PTSD, especially if there has been a head injury, are best treated with **Natrum Sulphuricum**.'

Dr Henry (psychiatrist): 'The new generation of antidepressants which cause an increase of serotonin in the brain are, in my opinion, extremely useful in the treatment of PTSD.'

Patrick (spiritual healer): 'In terms of trauma, if it's the wilful type, it goes to the very soul of the person and is the most difficult to integrate and heal. Accepting that incomprehensible things can be done to us at any time and that none of us are immune, is extremely difficult. When wilful trauma happens, a bubble of innocence is burst, leaving us stunned, dis-illusioned and feeling betrayed.

'From a spiritual perspective it takes an open heart chakra, with its energy of compassion and acceptance, to let go of a past hurt, to learn to value yourself again and get on with the business of rebuilding your life. For many this can seem like an impossible task. Trust has been broken and there is a feeling that a contract has been broken. 'This was not meant to happen to me. I didn't deserve it.' These seemingly random predicaments like rape, challenge us the most. Remaining open and vulnerable in an environment that is insecure and chaotic at times is not easy. What's the alternative — a closed heart and bunker living?

'Isabel's task, given that this horrific event has happened and cannot be reversed, is to either go under and live in perpetual fear, or to learn to trust again, which means risk-taking. She can stay trembling in the bunker or learn to feel secure in an insecure world. She's at a crossroads. Which way she goes will depend on the sum total of her past conditioning, both from this life and from past ones — i.e. her transpersonal programming, both conscious and unconscious, or her karma. It's this accumulated knowledge and wisdom that she will bring to bear on the direction she takes. Within the spiritual framework, it's not for anyone to judge whether or not she's taken the "right" path.'

CHAPTER 11 — Paranoia

Keynote: No Smoke Without Fire

Paranoia: Delusions of persecution, unwarranted jealousy, or an exaggerated sense of self-importance. A tendency to suspect and distrust others or to believe oneself to be unfairly used.   Oxford Dictionary

The way you see the world very much depends on your mind-set. We all have our own unique window on the world. Whatever currently pre-occupies you, you will literally see more of the same. If you are thinking of changing your car to a particular make, suddenly you will start seeing them everywhere. Of course they were always there; it is only now, because it matters to you, that you are noticing them. In this way we *co-create* the world we live in.

Whatever interests you — or is important to you at any point in time — seems to tune you in to any circulating information on that topic. We have all had the experience of having an 'out of the blue' synchronisation of events. You are in a bar and suddenly — coincidentally — you meet somebody who starts speaking about the same subject that you are working on at the moment. They have the one piece of information for which you were looking! Your antennae were scanning for that missing piece, it was on your mind and amazingly it materialises. At any other time it would not have registered, because it would not have been relevant — it would have passed over your head.

When you have been hurt, the most important thing in the world to you is to avoid a repetition. If you have been let down, betrayed or made a fool of, you have your antennae out for possible indications that it could happen again — this is your built-in watchdog. We are all paranoid about something!

If, on the other hand, you are doing something that you feel you should not be doing, you again have your antennae out. You want to avoid being found out and punished. If the tax on your car has expired, you will obviously suspect the worst from a passing police car. There is a tendency to over-personalise. If you are having an affair, you will be wary of your partner finding out. You may misinterpret your partner's innocent enquiry, 'So, where are you off to, all dressed up to kill?' Your 'guilt' colours the way you see things. You imagine a knowing tone in their voice, a raised eyebrow or a veiled threat, none of which are happening — or are they? Their remark, which would have been innocuous and irrelevant yesterday, suddenly sounds suspicious and significant today.

Paranoia — the word means 'beside your mind' from the Greek *para* (beside) and *noos* (mind) — is something of a bodyguard and in this sense is normal. Basically its vigilance has your interests at heart, but it can get out of control which happens when the fear levels are very high.

Patricia, a health board dentist, was investigated for fraud fifteen years ago. It was alleged that she was claiming payment for patients she had not seen. She strenuously fought the allegations, particularly since it had become public knowledge. Court proceedings both legal and ethical dragged on for four tortuous and stressful years. Getting off on a legal technicality, she knew she was fortunate not to have been found guilty, ending up instead with a token 'admonishment' from the dental ethics committee. One year ago she underwent a routine tax audit which brought up her worst fears, that she would be accused of fraud again. Having been caught with her hand in the cookie jar once, she naturally dreaded the same thing happening again.

Three months after the audit she had a visit from a health board official interviewing her with a view to funding an upgrade of her premises. She was tense during the meeting, feeling that it might be a cover to look at the actual running of her practice. Her suspicions grew when she got a phone call that afternoon from the same official proposing another meeting some weeks later to finalise details.

In the days that followed she started to believe that one of her patients was behaving in an over-inquisitive way, asking questions about the practice. *'Is he a plant, sent to spy on me?'* Two weeks later the phone service was disrupted for a number of hours, requiring a technician to check the internal lines. She interpreted this as a phone-tapping operation and even felt that a hidden camera might also have been installed. She kept her suspicions to herself, planning not to tell anybody until she had gathered sufficient evidence. She started to believe that anyone sitting in a car near her practice was monitoring her comings and goings and recording the number of patients attending her practice daily.

Married to a businessman, with three teenage children and a busy social life, on the surface Patricia's life went on as usual.

Nobody knew what she was thinking because she behaved in exactly the same way. Inside, however, the strain kept building and she became increasingly vigilant and on guard. Her racing thoughts kept her awake at night and she had a number of dreams in which she was being led away hand-cuffed to prison. When the health board official requested a postponement of the meeting she became alarmed. She saw it as a ploy to buy time, so that 'more' damning evidence against her could be collected.

When the meeting eventually took place she accused the official of spying on her. Surprised and taken aback he tried to reassure her, explaining in detail his real involvement, namely that of facilitating the funding for the renovations. Outraged at his 'cover up' she asked him to leave. On leaving the practice later she went straight to a police station to make a formal complaint and a statement was taken. As a result of the investigation which followed, she was notified by the health board to take immediate leave. She refused to co-operate and this led to her suspension pending a psychiatric assessment.

Scapegoating — Projecting Blame

At the core of paranoia is some extra-sensitivity to a past hurt. It may have been as a result of being two-timed in a relationship, publicly found out to have done something underhand or being passed over for a well-deserved promotion. Obviously where we have been hurt, our vigilant antennae are scanning for evidence of a possible 'hit' from the same source again. If you have had your heart broken, naturally you will be watchful in your new relationship. If you have been reprimanded by your boss for moonlighting while on sick leave, you will be doubly careful if you do it again so that you will not be caught. This makes good sense, but becomes a curse if it takes on exaggerated proportions as in Patricia's case.

If Patricia does not come to terms with her excessive paranoia through psychotherapy and other interventions, it may become hard-wired and written in stone. When this occurs the rigid mindset increasingly sees and filters the world in a biased way. *This distortion of reality is called a delusion, a false impression or interpretation not shared by others.*

In panic and anxiety there is a mounting sense of tension, an ominous dread of something awful about to happen which you have no way of controlling. Eventually you find from experience that if certain conditions are met, your inner turmoil eases. If you avoid certain places and things, such as shopping malls and spiders, you can feel more in control — and therefore 'safe'. A phobia has been born, you have found a scapegoat.

Similarly, in paranoia sufferers the sense of internal chaos which the original hurt creates is reduced by placing the cause outside themselves — there it becomes manageable. They feel that if they can avoid contact with the perceived source by 'boxing it off', they can get on with the rest of their lives. Their delusion gives them a sense of control and safety; but it becomes a real problem when the box can no longer contain it and explodes. Then it spreads, like a virus in a computer, to every aspect of the sufferers' lives.

In Patricia's case psychotherapy could help by encouraging her to trace the roots back to the source of her original hurt, the shame of having been caught 'fiddling'. There is never smoke without a fire. She interpreted this as a social death and was traumatised by it but never worked it through, instead she buried it and busied herself with her professional and family life. Thus she put it out of her mind and beyond her awareness into her unconscious — off the desktop and into the hard-drive.

Patricia's 'on the run' behaviours and distractions resulted from not integrating the experience at the time. When the additional stress of the tax audit came in, also carrying the theme of potential wrongdoing, she reached overload and could contain the tension no more.

Whenever there is too much material to download into consciousness without the system crashing, energetically the sixth chakra (see Appendix) comes to the rescue. This chakra, our 'third eye', is the centre where we interpret information and come up with solutions. It offloads the excess by projecting the problem back to the outside where it all started. This strategy pays off as it frees up energy to keep the rest of the system ticking over. On the surface the sufferer's life can continue as normal. However, if this projection continues over time, the subject it is projected onto will start reacting — a backlash inevitably follows. In Patricia's case she got herself suspended by falsely accusing the official with delusional information. In a self-fulfilling prophecy she is now under investigation, only this time for real! Everything gets so convoluted when it reaches this stage. Fact and fiction become intertwined and enmeshed.

Paranoia in the Schizophrenic State

Paranoid thinking can occur as a result of a schizophrenic break. What individuals experience in this boundless, altered state of consciousness is interpreted as frightening, bad, evil and persecutory. The interpretation is a reflection of the beliefs and values within their prior mindset. One individual sees God at work in the boundless experience, while another individual sees the hand of Satan. One feels saved and elevated, the other feels condemned and damned.

To complicate matters, *such can be the shifts of paranoid thought and its accompanying chemistry that auditory hallucinations can occur*. 'You're bad, you'll do harm to people, if you do that you'll be damned. You're being followed, you deserve to go to prison.' The voices can reflect the supposed wrongdoing and can frequently come in the form of recognisable people — a stern parent, teacher or other authority figures. Sufferers' self-loathing thoughts about themselves are echoed in actual audible voices. Diana, an English girl spending time on a small Greek island as an au pair, began a relationship with a local married man. They moved in together, to the disapproval of the village. He later moved back in with his wife — Diana was devastated, feeling betrayed and humiliated. She returned home under immense strain. The following week she began hearing voices, those of the old men in the village, calling her names and chastising her, not in her native English but in Greek.

Some musical composers actually hear the music playing in their head, an entire symphony, down to the last note. Beethoven's best music was written after he had already gone deaf. He had, in the course of his lifetime, created the necessary energetic and chemical pathways for hearing music in his head — that was his true musical genius. He was able to continue composing in spite of hearing loss.

The voices heard by a person in an altered state of consciousness appear to be an amplification of their thoughts. There is a link between the voices they 'hear' and past issues. Those promiscuous in the past may hear 'you're a whore', for example. This is an extreme case of the mind's ability to cross-reference. *Pathways already laid down dictate what they are likely to hear.* If all their life the internal conversation has been self-judging and self-loathing, they will be more likely now to hear 'voices' with that kind of content.

CHAPTER 12 — THE BROKEN H.

Keynote: Loss of the Believing Mirror

DANCE ME TO YOUR BEAUTY
WITH A BURNING VIOLIN
DANCE ME THROUGH THE PANIC
TILL I'M GATHERED SAFELY IN
LIFT ME LIKE AN OLIVE BRANCH
AND BE MY HOMEWARD DOVE
DANCE ME TO THE END OF LOVE

LEONARD COHEN

Romantic love, typified in Leonard Cohen's song is a state which, once experienced, is never forgotten. When we are in love our identity immediately changes. We let down the barriers of separateness, allowing ourselves to merge totally with the other. Perceived from the inside there is the experience of oneness, harmony, trust, unconditional love, acceptance, perfection, innocence, expansiveness and bliss.

The experience of love overrides other considerations such as duty, power, money, status and threat — no risk is too great. Nothing else matters but being together. Belief in the other is absolute. The fused energy and chemistry creates a world of its own. We positively 'glow' with health, on a physical, emotional and mental level. This expansion of energy allows us to express ourselves creatively, to enthusiastically embrace the world and relate to others compassionately. 'All the world loves a lover.'

Falling in love offers us the experience of having a *believing mirror* held up to us by the loved one. As we look into this mirror, features of ours are pointed out and admired, which we previously may not have recognised. We come to believe we are attractive, lovable, worthwhile and desirable. This feedback gives us confidence, self-esteem, a future and a sense of belonging. With our lover we co-create a new personal identity.

The loss of such love and our new way of defining ourselves, for whatever reason, can have an earthquake-like impact. Having tasted bliss, in its absence, we are worse off than we could ever have imagined. We are now living our worse nightmare. What is often not understood is that it is more than just the lovers presence that we miss, but the way we had come to feel about ourselves as part of that unit. *The 'self' that we had constructed in the presence of the other no longer exists — it has collapsed.* The self that had found an ultimate partner, the self whose future was secure and taken as a given, the self who was sexually irresistible, is no more. Our identity has died. It is the end. There is no future for it.

Between lovers there are *two* parallel relationships — lover to lover (interpersonal) and each lover to themselves (intrapersonal). When romance dies, there are therefore two deaths — one public and one private. The private death (the loss of the believing mirror) is little understood, difficult to articulate and can drive us mad.

Core issues instantly surface, such as abandonment, rejection, betrayal of trust and loss of control. This state of groundlessness is equivalent to the experience of the 'rug being pulled' from under us. Like a kite no longer held, we are cut adrift. Fear, anxiety and panic prevail and escalate when attempts to reattach prove futile.

BROKEN MIRROR, BROKEN HEART, BROKEN CORDS, BROKEN MIND

More men, women and, especially, adolescents have become insane in the wake of unrequited love affairs than those driven mad by toxins, defective genes and other abnormalities put together.

Edward M. Podvoll M.D.

Like one possessed, grieving lovers will describe the constant presence of the absent lover in their mind. We can think of nothing else. We become obsessed. We ruminate over and over how it ended, the reasons that put it beyond repair and what we could have done to prevent it. Imprisoned and haunted by all-pervading images and overwhelmed by our feelings, it becomes impossible to engage the outside world. Unable to concentrate, retain information, carry out simple tasks, maintain appearances, we become detached and indifferent. The world literally passes us by. These consequences accumulate and await us.

We have formed a relationship and built a life with a *memory,* rather than the real flesh and blood person. The energy connections or cords, chakra to chakra (see Appendix), which

were established during the relationship, have now been severed. Like phantom limbs we still feel their presence. Broken
cords translate into certain predictable behaviours. Demented,
like addicts in the height of withdrawal, we crave the loved
one's smell, their touch, their presence, everything about them.
To make matters worse, we idealise them and adore the ground
they walked on. We would do anything to reconnect and get
the 'fix'.

The relationship is lived out through any activity that keeps
it alive to us — visiting familiar haunts, rereading letters, looking at photographs and compulsively talking about the loved
one to whoever will listen. Anything to keep our old identity in
place — anything.

Like the bereaved, our grief goes through stages. We deny
it is over. We run through possible strategies to get them back,
plotting and planning, recruiting the support of accomplices,
seeking miracles, selling our soul. We vent our anger at ourselves, our ex-lover, their new lover, God or whoever. Unable
to control our thoughts we find our mind parasitised — no let-
up. We experience flashbacks during the day and our sleep is
broken by nightmares.

Obsessed by our mental turmoil, panic-stricken we ride an
emotional roller coaster. Behaving out of character we have 'lost
the run of ourselves' and descend into madness. We lose weight,
withdraw socially, rant and rave, weep, break things, drive dangerously, disappear for days, binge on drink and drugs, neglect
responsibilities and have thoughts of killing ourselves — our
condition resembles a Post-traumatic Stress Disorder.

We slide into the black hole of despair as we lose the grip
on our previous identity. Finally we realise that the believing
mirror is broken. More pathological expressions of these stages
can take the form of delusions, blackmail, stalking, crimes of
passion, psychosis and suicide.

OPEN HEART THERAPY

In our society is there a place to bring the broken heart for
healing? In times past and in different cultures, the expertise
of the shaman, the medicine man or the holy man might have
been sought. These days, if it is brought anywhere, it is brought
to the physician or the psychiatrist. It is the symptom that is presented, rarely the cause itself. The broken heart is in disguise,

in a distorted form. It is expressed as irritable bowel, headaches, insomnia, chest pain, asthma, chronic fatigue syndrome, substance abuse, depression, panic attacks, anxiety and suicidal attempts.

The real conversation is rarely engaged in because the focus of medicine is on symptom eradication. Within this framework, time is not allocated to what is causal — namely thoughts, meanings, values, emotions, energetic connections, sexual longings, self-worth etc. Society as a whole is intolerant of the bleeding heart beyond an arbitrarily set *heal-by date*. While the band-aid approaches offered by psychiatrists in the form of medication may have value in the short term with respect to restoring sleep, dampening down panic and energising mood, in the long term it is counterproductive, as psychotherapy is clearly indicated.

Gillian, a 26-year-old aspiring actress, was swept off her feet by Marty who was a talented director in fringe theatre. A passionate love affair ensued in which, for the first time ever, she felt valued and lovable. He called her a goddess and she revelled in her new-found sexuality. A stunningly beautiful man, heads would turn when he entered a room. Gillian, who regarded herself as 'plain' looking, began to look equally beautiful. She dressed extrovertly and received compliments that they made a striking couple. They worked together on a number of theatrical projects. It was the first time she felt that she had real talent as an actress. An outsider all her life, who had always found it hard to make friends, she suddenly found herself the centre of a huge social circle.

A year into the relationship, Gillian got a leading role in a play. The rehearsals took her over and their time together was limited. She went on tour with the company. On her return, he told her that he had fallen in love with her best friend. He rationalised his behaviour by accusing her of being wrapped up in herself and emotionally unavailable. This came like a bolt from the blue as he had always seemed supportive and to understand her commitments because he was in the same business.

Decimated, Gillian dropped everything and returned in panic to her home town and the safety of her parents house. Inconsolable in her grief she took to her bed. Any attempt by her parents to talk about it would reduce her to tears. Such was her mental turmoil that her parents had her referred to a psychiatrist. After trials of different medication she slid deeper and deeper into depression.

After six months she found that sympathy toward her was diminishing. Pressure was put on her to 'snap out of it'. The usual clichés were trotted out — get a life, forget about him, he is not worth it, there are plenty of fish in the sea. She hid the way she was feeling realising that they were all tired if it. Feeling isolated and lonely, Gillian began to anaesthetise her feelings with alcohol and medication.

G illian's experience is like a bereavement and is typical of a broken heart. Unlike in death, however, the elements of rejection and betrayal are in the forefront. The issue of 'not being good enough' does not have to be dealt with when a loved one dies. The object of her love is still alive, continuing his work, socialising in the same places and happily living with her best friend. To avoid the pain of ever meeting them she uprooted herself and fled to the last place she expected she would ever end up, at home, living with unsympathetic parents. Her loss is far greater than it would seem on the surface. Without the believing mirror, she no longer feels like a goddess, beautiful, sexually desirable, intelligent, witty, etc. — her identity has died. Resurrecting a new one seems to her an impossible task.

With bereavement there is a recognised ritual which provides healing time and allows for withdrawal from the pressures of the world. Support and shoulders to cry on are not in short supply. Not so with the broken heart, *where the healing process may even take longer.*

If we take a metaphysical approach to a broken heart and see it as a predicament, then the focus changes. Instead of focussing on the loss and its impact, it looks to what skills are required to be engaged so that an opportunity for resolving it becomes possible. It is obvious that new thoughts have to be created in order to replace the old ones — or at least suspend the old ones during the healing process — in this way a climate of learning is created. A healing listening space emerges in which support is given, in which there is an opportunity to be heard and feelings validated. Exploration of all the aspects of one's identity, relationship styles, issues of self-worth, abandonment, co-dependency and rejection can take place.

An energetic therapist may help identify blocks in the movement of energy (the chakras most affected by the crisis) and make the necessary interventions. The heart chakra is the centre of self-love and acceptance and without these there can be no healing. Self-loathing, criticism, mistrust and imbalance at all levels are the result. A homeopath might recognise the states of Ignatia, Natrum and Staphysagria and prescribe a remedy.

Heart energy in all spiritual traditions is seen as a central theme. *While religion relates to texts, spirituality relates to love.* At the core of Buddha and Christ consciousness lie the heart qualities of forgiveness, acceptance, peace and self-love. The heart is the centre of the chakra system, its purpose no different.

In Chinese medicine the mind is seen as residing in the heart and being responsible for different mental activities namely: thinking, memory, consciousness, insight, cognition, sleep, intelligence, wisdom and ideas.

A broken heart is not a trivial state. Look at it when it is open and active and you know what is missing. Living through your heart, you inhabit a different planet to those living it through their head. A person whose heart is closed is dead to themselves and the world.

ABSENCE OF A BELIEVING MIRROR — HEARTLESS CHILDHOODS

From the very moment of conception onwards through childhood, many people can find their presence rejected and invalidated. For whatever reason, no-one holds up a believing mirror to them. The focus is on their faults and their negative qualities, to such an extent that they feel their presence is an irritation and they are unwanted. This rejection is internalised by the child as the true reflection of their worth and they hold themselves responsible for being so flawed and for even existing at all.

Since they have never been perceived as lovable, they do not know how to love themselves or others. They live lives very much removed from the beautiful affirmation 'I am love, I am loving, I am lovable, I am loved.' Their heart chakra energy has never been encouraged to develop as it would under normal conditions, like a seed which has not germinated. A climate of fear, neglect and abuse is always anti-growth. In this way the heart chakra remains protectively closed.

Closed hearts express themselves later on in life as the endless list of dysfunctional adults engaging in addictions, child abuse, violence and other crimes against humanity. Bearing witness to this are the human products of institutional abuse, which was carried out under a wilful regime of unbridled brutality and sexual abuse, in orphanages, industrial schools and other such institutions.

A lesser known group of closed-hearted children emerge from families where love was conditional. Often middle class, with no shortage of material necessities, love was rationed. In the name of producing a child who would 'do their family proud', they are exposed to a regime of stick and carrot — approval is given only when the right standards are met. The self was reflected back only through the *parental mirror*. 'Kellys always come to the top of the pile.' 'There will be no gays in this house!'

With no firm sense of their own intrinsic value, they must perpetually seek it outside themselves. The opinions of others become their mirror, without it they have no identity. They relate to life as a survival exercise, accumulating by whatever means the trappings of external success — as if their life depended on it. In a sense it does.

IF MY HEART COULD DO MY THINKING
AND MY HEAD BEGAN TO FEEL
I WOULD LOOK UPON THE WORLD ANEW
AND KNOW WHAT'S TRULY REAL.

VAN MORRISON

SECTION 3

CHAPTER 13 — PSYCHOTHERAPY

Keynote: Soul Attendance

Strictly speaking, the question is not how to get cured, but how to live.
Joseph Conrad

Psychotherapy is a science which is as old as humanity itself. It derives from the Greek *psyche* meaning 'soul' and *therapeia* meaning 'attendance'. These days it has become associated with various schools of thought, disciplines, styles and approaches. Much has been written on the therapeutic relationship, strategic interventions, family and systemic dynamics, personality development, the role of past experience and the unconscious etc. Akin to designer styles and labels, famous names abound: Freud, Jung, Erickson, Adler, Rogers, Perls, Kelly, Lang, Lacan and Minuchin to name but a few.

It is beyond the scope of this book to explore the vast world of psychotherapy, comparing and contrasting the similarities and differences between styles, or to offer specific treatment strategies. This was never our aim: instead we have tried to keep the focus on the deeper significance of psychological distress and its relationship with our soul-purpose or spiritual dimension.

Due to the fact that the modern day doctor has inherited the mantle of the absent shaman, wise elder, seer or medicine man; the symptoms of disquiet, distress, unhappiness and problems of living are going to be interpreted through his or her professional mindset. In consequence, these symptoms are pathologised and as such become the enemy to be eradicated as quickly as possible. By 'shooting the messenger' in this way, the deeper origin of the disturbance is missed. The end result of this current approach, where the metaphysical contribution is ignored, is to reduce the human being to no more than biochemical soup. Such a reductionist view dis-empowers the individual, imprisons the mind, freezes the spirit and prevents any further learning — soul on ice!

Doctors and other professionals find themselves inadvertently engaging in 'fire fighting' roles, dealing with problems which present as medical, but whose origins lie in socioeconomic areas. How can a visit to a psychiatrist be expected to make someone more comfortable about their imminent redundancy? How can the distress of years of sexual abuse be easily

smoothed over and 'normal' life commenced? How can a worker not coping with the excessive demands within a multinational
company be adequately eased by a small white tablet? How can
a psychiatrist be expected to put the 'spark' back into a twenty-
five-year marriage in which coldness and feelings of rejection
abound? How can an educational psychologist change the competitive schooling system in which students are experiencing
ever-increasing levels of anxiety, occasionally accompanied by
suicidal thoughts?

The symptoms of intense distress, by their very nature, are
experienced in the present. Likewise, their relief is urgently
sought *now* — a quick fix is expected. The real solutions, however, often lie in the moderate to distant future. Child-oriented
social practices, a change in the school system, health and safety legislation in the workplace, redistribution of wealth and
essential resources are inevitably long-term solutions. The 'great
expectations' placed on the medical profession to deal with our
distress at life's setbacks is a titanic burden.

In the short term, doctors can offer empathy and some
relief. With the best will in the world, particularly in the area of
psychological medicine, hurried and superficial interventions
put in place because of the urgency of the symptoms may in the
long term generate dis-illusionment and cause further distress
when they do not work. The notion that all pain, all suffering
and all symptoms can be erased and life normalised is an
unhelpful illusion for either doctor or patient to have. Doctors
would be wise to display in their clinics the serenity prayer.

> GOD GRANT ME THE SERENITY
> TO ACCEPT THE THINGS I CANNOT CHANGE,
> THE COURAGE TO CHANGE THE THINGS I CAN
> AND THE WISDOM TO KNOW THE DIFFERENCE.

We see madness as one way individuals have of communicating their distress and their needs, a way which offers a solution of sorts to their dilemma. The work of a soul-attending
psychotherapist is to 'get behind' the symptom, decode its message and help sufferers to find a healthier way of getting their
needs heard than through the language of madness.

Psychotherapy in its broadest possible understanding reflects
a way of life. Having a spiritual perception alters everything. It
colours irreversibly how we relate to ourselves, those around us
and the world at large. It puts some kind of framework on some
of the more unsettling questions that make distress difficult to

bear like: 'Why me? Why now?' This perception brings with it no guarantees of happiness and success. It may even raise more questions than answers but it certainly pushes the envelope and opens up new horizons. Nothing appears as it seems any longer — everything is up for questioning. It is only in this place that the scientists, the mystics and the mad can sit down together and make sense of each other.

Exploring the territories of where life-purpose and soul-purpose overlap must be one of the most exciting of all human endeavours. The Great Mysteries can only await us: 'Who am I? Why am I here? Where am I going?'

By looking behind the scenes at the real-life characters of Mary, John, Julian, Carmel and others and their experiences of madness, we have gained an understanding of some of the threads woven into their distress. Through the voices of the panel we have tried to express a variety of causes and interpretations of these characters' problems, pointing to possible avenues of healing. In so doing we hope to impart to you, the reader, just how complex psychological distress can be in terms of the factors which contribute to it.

However, the healing process through psychotherapy can be made extraordinarily simple, if it meets three basic needs: *safety*, *self-love* and *a good reason to go on*. There is no psychotherapy particular to madness, only the *soul-attending* of individual human beings.

ALL DAY I THINK ABOUT IT, THEN
AT NIGHT I SAY IT.
WHERE DID I COME FROM AND
WHAT AM I SUPPOSED TO BE DOING?
I HAVE NO IDEA.
MY SOUL IS FROM ELSEWHERE,
I'M SURE OF THAT,
I INTEND TO END UP THERE. THIS DRUNKENNESS BEGAN
IN SOME OTHER TAVERN. WHEN I GET BACK AROUND
TO THAT PLACE, I'LL BE
COMPLETELY SOBER. MEANWHILE,
I'M LIKE A BIRD FROM ANOTHER
CONTINENT, SITTING IN THIS AVIARY.
THE DAY IS COMING WHEN I FLY OFF,
BUT WHO IS IT NOW IN MY EAR,
WHO SINGS MY VOICE?
WHO SAYS WORDS INTO MY MOUTH?
WHO LOOKS OUT WITH MY EYES?
WHAT IS MY SOUL?
I CANNOT STOP ASKING.

IF I COULD TASTE ONE SIP
OF AN ANSWER, I COULD BREAK OUT
OF THIS PRISON FOR DRUNKS.

I DIDN'T COME HERE OF MY OWN ACCORD,
AND I CAN'T LEAVE THAT WAY.
WHOEVER BROUGHT ME HERE
WILL HAVE TO TAKE ME HOME.

RUMI

Rumi's words resonate with an all too common experience summed up by *'What am I supposed to be doing? I have no idea.'* Without such answers we might find ourselves joining a queue to climb a ladder which is against the wrong wall! Rumi's lines *'My soul is from elsewhere, I'm sure of that, I intend to end up there,'* reflect a vague sense of spiritual longing somewhere in the recesses of our awareness. Rumi is asking basic questions. Which voice should we be listening to, the voice of our soul or the voice of our carefully constructed social reality? *'If I could taste one sip of an answer, I could break out of this prison for drunks.'*

ANATOMY OF CONSCIOUSNESS — A DIAGNOSTIC ROADMAP

If we understand psychotherapy to mean 'attending the soul' the next obvious question has to be, 'Where is the soul to be found?' We see the chakra system (see Appendix) and the energy field as a storehouse in which is encoded the knowledge gained from all the experiences we have ever had, including past lifetimes —also containing the template for our future lives with free will factored in. In Christian theology the trinity of the Father, Son and Holy Ghost is synonymous with the Life-force, the Physical Body and the Chakra System.

This system is communicating with us all the time through our thoughts, emotions, behaviours and physical status. Take the 'butterflies in the stomach' scenario before an examination. You feel afraid you will fail, are convinced you have not done enough work and would give anything to avoid being there — this is all third chakra language. If your energy continues to operate like this on a day-to-day basis for whatever reason, you will get a peptic ulcer, panic attacks, lose confidence or develop performance phobias. Symptoms at whatever level — be it mind, body or spirit — can be traced to the workings of the chakra system, whether it be a heart attack, cancer or a schizophrenic state.

The practice of psychotherapy has the potential to deal with all these dimensions of consciousness. These energy centres can function like a roadmap for therapist and client. It points to the location of certain issues, directs the way to their cause, offers signposts that tell us when balance has been lost and guides us toward resolutions. Each centre is best seen as having its own consciousness, its own personality, drives, needs and role within the system as a whole.

There is much mystique about the chakras. Even the name sounds strange to our western ears. The fact that they are invisible to most people certainly does not make them very accessible. However, in this sci-fi technological age, we are asked to take more and more for granted, especially if we cannot see it. Being unable to see the Web doesn't prevent us from accessing it.

Many who work in the bioenergy disciplines have an ability, through higher sense perception (verified for some time by scientific instrumentation), to see and feel the chakras. They see the electromagnetic energy field around the body as auras. They can therefore work directly with this energy by removing blocks and making possible the natural flow of life-force energy again.

The misunderstanding is that this higher sense perception is necessary in order for anyone to utilise its knowledge. All therapists, whether they know it or not, are working ultimately with the consciousness of each and every chakra at some level. (So are physicians, surgeons and the entire healing community.)

The scientific community have given us an understanding of quantum consciousness as the life-force behind everything, the interchangeability of wave and particle as well as absolute interconnectedness. They have taken us beyond real time and space. They even speak in spiritual language. What it has not done is given this knowledge a home within the self, a location where it can reliably be accessed and used. The chakra system is such a home.

HEALING THROUGH TIME DIMENSIONS

There is an increasing awareness, particularly through the work of Dr Brian Weiss and others, that psychotherapy needs to incorporate the knowledge of past lives and their influence on the present. We have worked both personally and professionally with spiritual healers who have provided us with another map with which to understand otherwise baffling phenomena. We have decided to represent this framework through the eyes of Patrick, the spiritual healer, on our panel of experts. What follows is a case example in which leakage from a past life was central to the lack of resolution of a problem.

Jack was a sixteen year old with two elder sisters, from as early as the parents could remember he had had problems with his temper. He was irritable, grumpy, sullen, unco-operative and could never be criticised. If he was challenged he would fly into a rage, break things, kick people, scream and use abusive language. Although socially skilled and with no shortage of friends he constantly fell out with them and, as a result, was being marginalised. He mainly reserved his venom for his family and no matter what they did to try to win him over, he remained unchanged. Discipline made him worse. His parents good-humouredly referred to him as the 'child from hell' and pondered where he had come from.

Family psychotherapy was of no avail as he refused to own his part in the problem. It was always somebody else's fault. His sisters walked around him as if on eggshells, aware that even breathing 'the wrong way' could set him off. The family were held to ransom by his behaviour.

His mother consulted with a spiritual healer and taped the session. According to his reading Jack was miscarried in his last lifetime when his mother fell drunk down a stairway. That entity was prevented from completing the life he had planned with that mother. 'I see the entity looking at that mother with another child in her arms and saying over and over that it should have been him.'

He explained that Jack's anger was because he felt he should never have come into his present family. He observed that his energy was mostly absent from the lower chakras. Jack felt outraged at this abandonment and his heart chakra remained closed much of the time. He was using his sixth to justify his self-righteous behaviour. Patrick saw his karmic task now as one of learning to accept this incarnation and to trust again.

His mother had told Jack that she was going to talk to a 'psychic' and he was strangely curious and interested. When she played him the tape he listened intently and to her surprise began to sob inconsolably. He told her that he always felt like he didn't belong in the family, even believing that he was adopted. He felt relieved that there was an explanation for his temper because he hated himself for being like that, but could not seem to help it.

The spiritual healer recommended that Jack needed to cut the energetic cords with his past-life mother. This he did and practiced the exercises necessary to complete that process. In the following weeks there was a noticeable improvement in Jack's behaviour. After six months he became calm and began to enjoy family life.

We are all familiar with the difference a framework of explanation makes, whether it is making sense of a worrying symptom or finally figuring out to where your passport has disappeared. Once we know what we are dealing with, that seems to point to a solution all by itself.

The quantum physicists tell us that the past, present and future time dimensions all occur at once. This is confusing because our limited consciousness cannot understand. We have all had déjà vu experiences, premonitions and dreams that predict future events — these are examples of leakage between the time dimensions. Clairvoyants have the capacity to voluntarily expand their consciousness so that they can 'see' events happening in different space-time dimensions. The direct vivid experience of a past life with all the sensory information intact, through hypnosis, holotropic breathwork and other means, is becoming increasingly commonplace.

Medicine is on the cusp of a new paradigm. The imminent leap is equivalent to that which physics has already made, namely moving from the Newtonian to the Quantum age. Larry Dossey M.D., a forerunner in the exploration of the crossroads of spirit and physical health, describes three medical eras:

- Era I – where all forms of therapy are focussed solely on the effect of things on the body, and where mind is not a factor in healing, dominated medicine from the late 1900s, until about 1950, but is still influential.
- Era II – the era of mind–body medicine, where mind has causal power, and therapies emphasise the effect of

consciousness on healing, includes but goes beyond Era I, and is not fully explainable by classical concepts in physics.

- **Era III** – non-local or transpersonal medicine, includes therapies in which effects of consciousness bridge between different persons, and in which mind is seen as unbounded and infinite in space and time. These are not describable by classical concepts of space–time or matter–energy.

Medicine is on the threshold of an expansion from a mind–body focus (Era II) to embrace the dimension of spirit (Era III). An increasing knowledge of the chakra system, the influence of past life experiences and the place for distant healing is evidence that that expansion has begun. Like the shift from flat-earth to round-earth consciousness, our scientific validation of the new consciousness must keep up. Why should medicine be concerned with these newly documented phenomena? In Larry Dossey's own words:

> The reason is straightforward: these events can and do affect the body in dramatic ways. I suggest that *anything* that significantly affects the functions of the body . . . is the legitimate concern of medicine.

EPILOGUE

In the book and movie *The Cider House Rules*, the story pivots around the central theme of acceptance and non-judgement. A set of rules which are posted up on the wall of the cider house, the barn in which the seasonal apple-pickers live, creates the metaphor around which the drama unfolds — whose message is live and let live. The cider house rules were made by the owners, who did not have to live there. They were regarded by the workers as ridiculous because they had nothing to do with the reality of their day-to-day living. Ironically, the behaviours that the rules prohibited, like smoking in bed and sitting on the roof, were the very things that made life there bearable!

As the story develops and various dilemmas present themselves, each of the main characters evolve their own set of personal 'rules'. We are drawn into the workings of their minds and the ways they choose to live their lives. All of them are prepared to take full responsibility for their actions and the effect they have on others.

From a very early age we all learn the rules and conditions we have to satisfy in order to be loved, gain approval and belong — our behaviours are either rewarded or punished. Most of us grow up with the sound of 'behave yourself' ringing in our ears. This does not imply behave like yourself, but rather according to the rules of others — there is a long list. The needs of parents, siblings, peers, teachers and other outsiders all have to be met.

The adult version of being 'in the club' and of the 'right stuff' is often at odds with who we are inside. It takes a lot of guts to break through the social constraints and do your own thing, in your own way. It has something to do with spontaneity, 'to be or not to be' and seizing the moment. This is not the stuff of revolution or anarchy, but much more in the style of Kevin Spacey's character in *American Beauty*, who wanted to simplify his life by chucking in his meaningless job in advertising and instead flip hamburgers in the local diner. A way of life which did not appeal to his wife's upwardly mobile view of success! Nonetheless he had the courage to go for it — he took the consequences.

BE YOUR OWN SCRIPTWRITER

At the core of mental well-being is the central issue of being authentic, which derives from the Greek *authentikos*, 'to be your own author' — to write your own script. While society pays lip-service to the notion of personal freedom and the right to do it your own way, it vociferously disapproves if you go outside its carefully prescribed 'rules'. If being yourself means inconveniencing others, creating a fuss, not meeting certain standards, showing vulnerability, being different or falling apart — there is a sharp intake of breath.

Battered wives, closeted gays, sexually frustrated priests, the abused, disgruntled employees, the panic stricken and the dis-illusioned all pay a high price for not 'coming out'. Shame, guilt and the stigma of being on the 'wrong' list act as a ball and chain, paralysing them with fear, locking them into inauthentic roles and stifling growth. In this territory, following your star is an illusion.

Years of clinical practice have made us aware of three states which are consistently present in the psychologically distressed, namely fear, self-loathing and a strong desire 'not to be here'. *Their presence is the very antithesis of well-being.* They evolve when any of us cannot meet the demands of imposed rules and conditions in order to have our basic needs met. How different our life would be if we did not have to surrender our individuality, bury our authenticity and fit into the mores of a fickle society.

We *learn* to be afraid. There is no gene for self-loathing. 'Not wanting to be here' sums up our sense of dis-illusionment: shattered dreams, broken promises.

As Heraclitus said, 'You never step into the same river twice.' Everything is in perpetual movement, constantly changing. No two seasons, no two days, no two hours are the same and so on. Yet we want them to be, because familiarity gives us a sense of security. The same applies to ideas, beliefs and attitudes. We want the known to remain the same, which is an impossibility. When change appears on the horizon and we do not feel equipped to deal with it, it becomes a predicament. It perplexes us and we see danger in the situation. It can fill us with fear and we wish it would go away. 'The last thing I needed was this!'

Psychological distress inevitably arises out of predicaments and the state of imbalance into which they throw us. Our reserves, skills, resources and coping strategies are called into question during such difficult times. In our culture, the mental and emotional equivalent of physical distress (such as pain) is pushed out of sight and out of mind. We loathe ourselves for being so weak and vulnerable. We are afraid to acknowledge to ourselves or anyone else that we are out of our depth and going under. Why is this?

If I could put my hand up and say 'I'm not waving, I'm drowning' and be greeted with enthusiastic support, how much freer I would feel to share my distress and how much safer. To hear 'No problem, it is temporary, we will stand by you, take as long as you need, there is plenty that can be done,' is hopeful and fosters security. This is very different from being looked at through professional goggles and hearing phrases trotted out like 'You have a chemical imbalance. It's genetic in origin. You'll have it for life. You'll need to stay on medication. You may have relapses.' It is back to cider house rules, where the outsider assumes they know what the insider needs.

BREAKING THE MOULD

FOR THIS SOUL NEEDS TO BE HONOURED WITH A NEW DRESS WOVEN
FROM GREEN AND BLUE THINGS AND ARGUMENTS THAT CANNOT BE PROVEN

PATRICK KAVANAGH

Psychiatry does not have a healing reputation. It rarely resonates with its Greek origins (*psyche* meaning soul, and *iatriea* meaning healing) or with the sentiment of the poet Patrick Kavanagh's plea for what the soul needs. For many the experience of hospitalisation is both traumatising and stigmatising, adding to the original distress. Some people on discharge are actually post-traumatically stressed. Others are overwhelmed by the news that they have a 'lifelong disease' and many leave with more fear than they came in with – certainly with more self-loathing.

The history of psychiatry is a horror story, and the fear of it remains deeply embedded in our collective unconscious, contributing to the stigma of psychological distress. Just because a style of practice has been in place for a long time does not make it right.

People say again and again that philosophy doesn't really progress, that we are still occupied with the same philosophical problems as were the Greeks. But the people who say that don't understand why this has to be so. It is because our language has remained the same and keeps seducing us into asking the same questions.   Wittgenstein

We hold that the same is true of psychiatry. It needs a new language, and to ask new questions.

Psychiatry practised as soul healing embraces the multi-dimensional nature of what it is to be human and puts the distress in its rightful place. The moment a suffering individual is seen as a mind–body–spirit organism on a journey through life, everything changes. Now it is a level playing field, human-to-human, expert-to-expert. Out of this therapeutic stance evolves a healing programme tailor-made with the insider's needs paramount. For some this may mean negotiating their way out of a dead-end job, ending a dysfunctional relationship, clearing debts and making a safe space in which to bring past hurts to the surface. Reality-based conversations may be needed with family members and employers, and other transformational services accessed to facilitate the smoothing of the path forward. None of this is necessary if it is all 'chemical'.

BITING THE BULLET

Each one of us has a duty to deal with what limits and constricts the quality of our lives and our future growth. Risks have to be taken, responsibility shouldered, support sought and a campaign mounted by us in the direction of change. Life is about our personal journey and whether or not we learn from the predicaments we encounter — nobody else can live it for us. We can seek out help and guidance but it is naïve to think that we can hand our mind, our body or our spirit over to professional bodies (be they legal, religious or medical) and believe that we will come back 'fixed'. There is no cavalry coming, no ultimate rescuer.

Life cannot wait until the sciences may have explained the universe sci-
entifically. We cannot put off living until we are ready. The most salient
characteristic of life is its coerciveness: it is always urgent, 'here and
now' without any possible postponement. Life is fired at us point-blank.
José Ortega y Gasset

Taking control of our lives and liberating ourselves from our
personal difficulties is essential if we decide not to see life
as a dress rehearsal. The transcendence of huge personal obsta-
cles by individuals such as Helen Keller, Christy Brown, Christopher Reeves, Jean-Dominique Bauby and Amelia Corry bear
witness to what lies within the human repertoire of possibility
once the spirit is ignited. They refused to lie down when life
was fired at them 'point-blank'.

However, in a climate of paralysing fear, all our energy goes
into staying safe. There is little available for pro-activity; in fact
we need 'cradling' and someone on whom to temporarily pass
the baton. There are seasons to the giving and receiving of help.
It is as inappropriate for someone who needs cradling to be
pressurised into pro-activity as it is for those easily capable of
being proactive to want to be spoon-fed.

Everything But the Kitchen Sink

If you have decided it is time to be proactive in your own healing, to swim rather than sink, keep at it until you have
reached the shore. This means continuing until you find a match
with a healing modality which suits you. A child experiences
pain relief when a band-aid is applied. Clinical trials reveal anything between twenty-five and seventy-five per cent improvement when a placebo or dummy drug is given in place of the
real thing. Belief in the healing you are being administered
accentuates the body's own natural resources. The body is its
own healer. It replicates millions of cells daily, repairs and
replaces damaged tissue and combats infection. Outside interventions merely piggyback onto this life-force already at work.

It is only when a mutual understanding is in place between
patient and doctor, client and counsellor, that healing can com-
mence in earnest. Fear, doubt and helplessness on the part of
the patient, matched with an absence of empathy and understanding on the part of the doctor, is the biggest obstacle to

healing. It has to be a co-operative effort. If either one party or the other are not synchronised, then there is no hope of change.

In the area of psychological distress, *intention and conscious choice-making are the most important ingredients in healing*. If your life is full of fear and you are hiding away in a bunker, filled with self-loathing, progressively constricting and withering, this will not change unless you come out and seek the cradling you need. You need to become a pilgrim in search of healing or you will end up miserable and helpless — a victim. We would encourage people to continue searching until the 'gel' is right with either their doctor or their treatment. If the medication is not working, take yourself off to a psychotherapist. If that does not work, go to a homeopath, an energy worker, an acupuncturist or a spiritual healer.

Activate your life-force and break the cycle. Energise your system by getting physically fit, doing yoga, by having massage and by eating and sleeping well. Remind your senses what they are for, by bringing in pleasure. Have fun, see friends, titillate your taste buds, listen to your favourite music, feast your eyes, burn essential oils, take long baths, dress yourself up, have sex — detoxify. Stop ingesting what you know very well is bad for you. Eliminate negative relationships, change jobs, make positive lifestyle changes. Share your problems with good listeners — connect to the tribe. Get skills, do self-development courses, take up a hobby and engage life actively. Spend time in nature, meditate and stimulate your brain.

Push the envelope, take risks, do whatever is necessary to break the cycle of misery, loneliness and victimisation. Visualise yourself well and happy. Healthy anticipations and intentions are powerful medicines. Appeal to the gods, spend time in an ashram, visit Lourdes or whatever. Take up your bed and walk, walk, walk. It is better to keep experimenting than to curl up in a ball, like a zombie in front of a TV, drugged up to your eyeballs, the psychiatric version of a couch potato. 'Cure me but don't change me.'

When your very soul (psyche) is hanging in the balance, there is no room for complacency. Seek clarification wherever you can find it — educate yourself. Search the Net, read; get second, third and fourth opinions if necessary. Do not be intimidated by the 'weight' of medical opinion. Let your own intuition be your guide.

There is obviously much more unknown knowledge than known. Innovation, tools for expanding consciousness are around the next corner. Discovery is not only the preserve of computer science, it is happening in the healing professions too. For example, who would have thought that a Harvard psychiatrist, Dr Brian Weiss, would have his belief system turned upside down by his unexpected discovery of the usefulness of past-life regression? It challenged him to see spirituality and healing sitting side-by-side; just like the Jackies, the Patricks and the Dr Clarkes on our panel. These are real people who exist in our professional world and who do invaluable work pushing the boundaries of healing. There is plenty more where they came from, all practising from a position of openness, hope, compassion, acceptance and the belief that Anything is Possible.

THE JOURNEY

ONE DAY YOU FINALLY KNEW
WHAT YOU HAD TO DO AND BEGAN,
THOUGH THE VOICES AROUND YOU
KEPT SHOUTING
THEIR BAD ADVICE —
THOUGH THE WHOLE HOUSE
BEGAN TO TREMBLE
AND YOU FELT THE OLD TUG
AT YOUR ANKLES.
'MEND MY LIFE!'
EACH VOICE CRIED.
BUT YOU DIDN'T STOP.
YOU KNEW WHAT YOU HAD TO DO,
THOUGH THE WIND PRIED
WITH ITS STIFF FINGERS
AT THE VERY FOUNDATIONS,
THOUGH THEIR MELANCHOLY
WAS TERRIBLE.
IT WAS ALREADY LATE
ENOUGH AND A WILD NIGHT,
AND THE ROAD FULL OF FALLEN
BRANCHES AND STONES.
BUT LITTLE BY LITTLE,
AS YOU LEFT THEIR VOICES BEHIND,
THE STARS BEGAN TO BURN
THROUGH THE SHEETS OF CLOUDS,
AND THERE WAS A NEW VOICE
WHICH YOU SLOWLY
RECOGNISED AS YOUR OWN,
THAT KEPT YOU COMPANY
AS YOU STRODE DEEPER AND DEEPER

INTO THE WORLD,
DETERMINED TO DO
THE ONLY THING YOU COULD DO —
DETERMINED TO SAVE
THE ONLY LIFE YOU COULD SAVE.

MARY OLIVER

APPENDIX — THE CHAKRA SYSTEM

Keynote: The Door to Vibrational Medicine

It is beyond the scope of this book to cover the chakra system in any great detail. The word chakra comes from the Sanskrit *cakra* meaning a wheel or circle. What follows is a brief outline of its basic principles.

As humans we are vibratory beings composed of matter and non-matter which co-exist at different frequencies, ranging from skin and bone to thoughts and feelings. Visible and invisible, material and non-material, all interconnected within our multidimensional anatomy.

When we hear a voice, we are not actually hearing it with our ears but in our consciousness. The hearing apparatus brings in the vibration created by the sound, which is interpreted, given meaning and 'heard' by the mind. The same is true of sight and the other senses. Our anatomical eye brings in the vibrating photons of light, which are then 'seen' within the matrix of our interpretations, beliefs, attitudes and conditioning, discriminating what is meaningful or not to our needs, wants and desires.

Everything that human beings have ever created, has had to first exist as a thought, a vibrating impulse of energy and information. In the outer world thoughts have put a man on the moon, painted the *Mona Lisa,* and masterminded the holocaust. In the inner world thoughts have the power to set in motion cascades of electrical impulses and neurochemicals, the endpoint of which is experienced by us as stillness, joy, love, hurt, health, madness, or dis-ease. The operational software of consciousness has limitless possibilities, offering us infinite choices, and endless creativity.

The vibratory frequencies of the physical body, its feelings, and its thoughts, are detectable as a surrounding energy field. It functions much like a lung, not only transmitting but also receiving, processing and integrating energy impacting on it. Temperature changes, noise levels, personal interactions, television, phone and radio waves, pollutants and even the movements of planets all flow through our energy field before they interface with the physical body.

Like a molecule of water within the larger ocean, we are inseparable from the vibrations that surround us, some of which

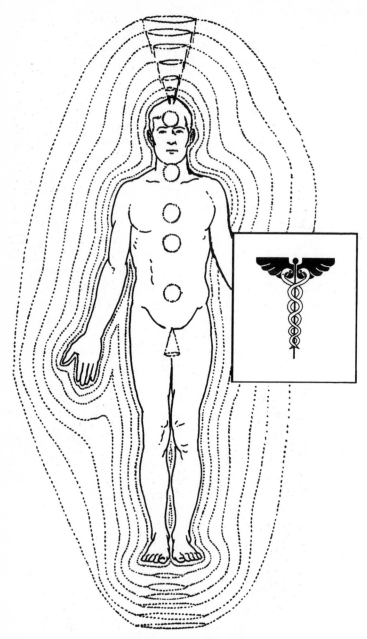

The Chakras and the Energy Fields

Inset — The caduceus, the symbol of healing used by modern medicine is based on the chakra system.

we perceive, most of which we don't. Our energy field is the permeable boundary which defines our sense of individuality. Quantum physics defines us as a localised organisation of consciousness within a conscious universe. We are not merely a speck in the eye of the universe but a thought in its mind.

The outermost layer of the energy field, referred to as the causal body, acts like a template or blueprint for the physical body, shaping such things as cellular development, specification, replication and repair. This template is there from our very beginning, when we start life as a fertilised egg evolving in 3-4 days into 32 non-differentiated cells. It is at this precise moment that a mind-boggling crescendo occurs — cellular specification. It poses the question. How does a bundle of tiny cells all identical and with equal potential for specialising into nerve cells, muscle cells, bone cells, skin cells etc. know what to do? (How does a nerve cell 'know' not to become a muscle cell?)

The answer lies at source, namely that the organisational intelligence resides not in the cells themselves but in the surrounding template. In other words the guiding force is contained within the energy field and imbues each cell with its personalised piece of vital information so that it can play its part in the composition of the whole. This is analogous to the participation of each individual musician in an orchestra collectively playing a symphony under the direction of a conductor.

The pattern of potential disease can be found as a disturbance in the energy field before it manifests in the body as pathology. In the emerging paradigm of quantum healing or vibrational medicine, diagnostics and treatment interventions will operate at the level of the energy field and the chakra system, building on the current use of ultra-sound, lasers and radiation. Vibrational practices already in place include the use of crystals, flower essences, homeopathic remedies, acupuncture, essential oils, colour and sound, prayer, meditation, bodywork, bio-energy and psychotherapy.

Incoming energies passing through the body's energy field are integrated into the cellular matrix by specialised step-down transformers known as the chakras. These are centres or vortices of electromagnetic energy found within the body at clearly definable anatomical positions. They are best seen as the primary sensory organ which processes higher electrical frequencies, outside the range of the other five senses, converting them into a wave pattern that can be utilised by the cells of the physical body.

Anatomically each chakra is associated with a major nerve plexus and endocrine gland. Together these create a regulatory control system which affects the physiology of the body, ranging from cellular gene activation, on up to the functioning of the central nervous system, and ultimately feeling and thought. In this way the chakras affect our moods and behaviours through hormonal influences on brain activity.

The seven major chakras run along the central axis of the body from the base of the spine to the crown of the head, and are interconnected with and inseparable from the energy field. Each can be seen as a floppy disc, which not only contains programmed sub-routines with memory updates, but receives new information, filters it, and transmits it to every cell and back out to the energy field. Each chakra is interconnected with the other six rather like an electro-magnetic circuit board. The bio-programme contained within each influences our cells, and shapes our thoughts, feelings, and behaviours. As such it can be seen as having its own distinct personality, emotional tone, psychological agenda, karmic and spiritual map.

It is through the chakra system and its intimate contact with the energy field, which is in turn in relationship with the universal mind, that the life-force or universal consciousness is mediated to us as individuals. This system is where karmic imprints are stored from previous lifetime experiences, and through which they are activated and expressed in the current lifetime.

THE SEVEN MAJOR CHAKRAS

The degree of harmony between the seven chakras influences the level of performance of every physical, emotional, mental and spiritual function of our mind-body-spirit organism. Such balance can depend on the degree of openness or closure at any given moment of an individual chakra or all of them.

Chakra imbalance frequently begins within a context of fear. This can happen following a range of life difficulties such as childhood traumas, physical pain, social conditioning, deprived and oppressive environments, mental and emotional shocks, prolonged stress and anything that constricts our unique personal consciousness and its full expression.

The **first chakra** is located at the base of the spine. The verb that best describes it is 'I have' or 'I exist'. Its primary role deals with the survival of our physical identity. My first chakra will tell me how much sleep I need, how much food to eat, how to find a place to live, a means of independent income, how to behave in the face of danger, and provides me with the means to be grounded in all aspects of my physical reality. It can be compromised in the face of survival issues and threats to existence. It vibrates at the red end of the colour spectrum.

The **second chakra** is located below the navel and its verb is 'I feel'. As the centre of my emotional intelligence it influences my ability to experience pleasure and to avoid pain, to respond to change, experience my sexuality and deal with the issues of intimacy, parenting, relationships and community. Its vibration is orange.

The **third chakra** is located in the solar plexus and its verb is 'I can'. It deals with individual identity, self-definition, ego strength and willpower — the ability to influence my life. Its issue is personal autonomy, 'fire in the belly' and is vital to the notion of standing on my own two feet. Its vibration is yellow.

The **fourth chakra** is located in the middle of the chest, behind the breastbone and its verb is 'I love'. It is through this chakra that we feel unconditional acceptance of ourselves, others, and reality as it is. Here dwells the ability to feel compassion, the drive towards harmony and peace, and the openness to give and receive. Its vibration is green.

The **fifth chakra** is located in the throat and its verb is 'I speak'. It helps me to express myself and explore my special talents, to be authentic to my true nature, hear other people empathically, put form on my ideas, and think symbolically. It is the centre associated with creativity and its vibration is sky blue.

The **sixth chakra** is located in the centre of the forehead and is metaphorically referred to as 'the third eye'. Its verb is 'I see'. It deals with insight, reflection, intuition, visualisation, values and beliefs, the realm of abstraction and the ability to see the bigger picture. Imbalance in the sixth chakra is reflected in the inability to see clearly, losing the plot, fragmentation, inflexibility, rigid belief systems, delusions, poor concentration, hallucinations, and nightmares. Its vibration is midnight blue or purple.

The **seventh chakra** is located at the crown of the head and is associated with the issues of self-knowledge, the higher self, spiritual understanding, a sense of divinity within, our connection to a higher power and our place in the grand design. The verb is 'I know' and the vibration is purple or white.

A Case Example of Chakra System Imbalance

Nancy, a forty-five-year-old married woman with two children, was involved in a fatal road traffic accident near her home. She was negotiating a traffic junction when an ambulance which was answering an emergency call hit her car broadside. Such was the impact that the car was literally lifted into the air and thrown into the front garden of a suburban house. The ambulance driver was killed. She sustained multiple fractures to her ribcage and both legs. She had an out-of-body experience where she looked down on herself being cut out of the car by the fire brigade.

In spite of gaining full mobility within a period of three months, eight months later she was still in emotional turmoil, and was diagnosed as suffering from post-traumatic stress disorder. In shock, frozen in time and not fully functioning in her daily reality, she felt dislodged from her previous ways of thinking, feeling and behaving. Nancy felt as though she was looking at life through a 'pane of glass'.

First chakra symptoms: She felt fatigued, demotivated, panicky, hypervigilant, vulnerable and had a sense of impending doom. With her sleep disrupted, she had little energy and felt that she was 'running on empty'.

Second chakra symptoms: She felt 'emotionally numb', got little pleasure from her pre-accident activities and behaviours, and lost interest in sex. She began sleeping apart from her husband. Feeling emotionally overwhelmed, she found it difficult to meet the demands of her two teenage children, responding with irritability or bouts of crying.

Third chakra symptoms: Previously confident and socially at ease, she now suffered from low self-esteem, lacked drive and confidence, and socially she withdrew. Her sense of loss of control over her life was expressed as panic attacks.

Fourth chakra symptoms: Nancy became her own worst critic and was impatient with her slow recovery. She kept blaming herself for her lack of progress, and was unable to feel the benefit of her family's efforts to support and love her. Her husband's affection seemed patronising. To her the world was an uncompassionate, unfair and harsh place. 'Why me?'

Fifth chakra symptoms: She felt unable to express her feelings and she frequently felt misunderstood by those around her. She held back from explaining her truly desperate situation for fear that she would be judged, misinterpreted or at worst mocked.

Sixth chakra symptoms: Constant vivid intrusive thoughts relating to the accident were in the forefront of her mind, which triggered flashbacks. She experienced accident-related nightmares and was afraid to drive the car. Her concentration and short-term memory were poor. She judged herself as being 'stupid'. Feeling she had lost the plot, she became disillusioned with life and wondered what was the point of it.

Seventh chakra symptoms: Feeling set apart from other people and disconnected from life she felt abandoned and alienated. 'If there was a God where is he now?'

This phenomenon of experiencing an energy shutdown is common in life-threatening experiences such as road-traffic accidents, assaults, rape, grief, or sudden loss. In addition it occurs in prolonged states of energy imbalance such as chronic fear, chronic depression and burnout. If this electromagnetic disturbance is not resolved, it ultimately leads to physical changes and disease.

A Reflection

Vibrational medicine invites us to embrace the holographic intelligence of the life-force, the presence of spirit in every wave and particle of our multidimensional anatomy and the correlation of cause and effect. It opens the door to healing at a quantum level, and places us in the witness position from where we can best see the effects of our thoughts, feelings, and behaviours on our mental and physical well-being.

THERE IS A BEING, WONDERFUL, PERFECT;
IT EXISTED BEFORE HEAVEN AND EARTH.
HOW QUIET IT IS!
HOW SPIRITUAL IT IS!
IT STANDS ALONE AND DOES NOT CHANGE.
IT MOVES AROUND AND AROUND, DOES NOT ON THIS ACCOUNT SUFFER.
ALL LIFE COMES FROM IT.
IT WRAPS EVERYTHING IN ITS LOVE AS IN A GARMENT, AND YET CLAIMS NO
     HONOUR, FOR IT DOES NOT DEMAND TO BE LORD.
I DO NOT KNOW ITS NAME, AND SO I WILL CALL IT TAO, THE WAY, AND REJOICE
     IN ITS POWER.

LAO-TZU

FURTHER READING

Bailey, Philip, M.D., *Homeopathic Psychology*, North Atlantic Books, CA 1995
* Portraits of the common constitutional remedies.

Barlow, David H., *Anxiety and its Disorders*, The Guildford Press, NY 1988
A scientific look at panic and anxiety.

Bourne, Edmund J., Ph.D., *The Anxiety and Phobia Workbook*, New Harbinger Publications Inc., CA 1990
An excellent practical DIY for stress and anxiety.

Brennan, Barbara Ann, *Hands of Light*, Bantam Books 1987
The most comprehensive study of hands-on healing.

Capra, Fritjof, *The Turning Point*, Simon and Schuster 1982
The bridge between quantum physics and mysticism.

Chopra, Deepak, *Quantum Healing*, Bantam Books 1989
The role of quantum consciousness in healing.

Chopra, Deepak, *The Seven Spiritual Laws of Success*, Bantam Press 1996
A masterpiece of spiritual writing. Seven simple steps to mind-body-spirit living.

Coelho, Paulo, *Veronika Decides to Die*, Harper Collins 1998
A novel which celebrates love as a transformative force in a psychiatric hospital.

Dossey, Larry, *Healing Words*, Harper, San Francisco 1993
A serious medical look at the healing power of prayer.

Francis, Patrick, *The Grand Design*, Auricle Books 1995
One psychic healer's map of the spiritual realm.

Gerber, Richard, M.D., *Vibrational Medicine*, Bear and Co., New Mexico 1998
A cutting edge tome on the emerging role of energy in medicine.

Goleman, Daniel, *Emotional Intelligence*, Bloomsbury, London 1996
Emotional IQ and its role in our personal evolution.

Grof, Christina and Stanislav Grof, M.D., *The Stormy Search for the Self*, Thorsons 1990
An interpretation of madness as a spiritual emergency.

Ingham, Christine, *Panic Attacks*, Thorsons 1993
An excellent DIY manual.

Jamison, Kay Redfield, *An Unquiet Mind*, Picador 1995
An insider's view by a psychologist who experienced mania.

Judith, Anodea, *Eastern Body — Western Mind*, Celestial Arts, CA 1996
The bible on the chakras and energy field and how they are expressed.

Kabat-Zinn, Jon, *Full Catastrophy Living*, Delacorte Press 1990
  An accessible read on bringing meditation into everyday life.
Kornfield, Jack, *The Path With Heart*, Bantam/Doubleday Dell 1993
  A heartfelt look at meditation with many beautiful exercises.
Matsakis, Aphrodite, Ph.D., *Post Traumatic Stress Disorder*, New
  Harbinger Publications, CA 1994
  An academic look at post traumatic stress.
Miller, Alice, *The Drama of Being a Child*, Virago 1983
  *This little gem looks at the damage done when our inner child
  is silenced.*
Myss, Caroline, Ph.D., *Anatomy of the Spirit*, Bantam Books 1997
  Examines the spiritual symbolism of the chakra system.
Pert, Candace, Ph.D., *The Molecules of Emotion*, Simon and Schus-
  ter, London 1997
  *A scientific explanation of how our feelings are chemically
  created.*
Podvoll, Edward, M.D., *The Seduction of Madness*, Harper Collins,
  NY 1990
  Chronicles of the journey into mania.
Watson, J. Allen, M.D., *The Chemistry of Conscious States*, Little
  Brown and Co. 1994
  *A highly readable book on the chemistry that drives con-
  sciousness.*
Weiss, Brian, M.D., *Many Lives, Many Masters*, North Atlantic
  Books, CA 1995
  *A psychiatrist's introduction to past lives through one patient's
  experience under hypnosis.*
Zohar, Danah and Dr Ian Mitchell, *Connecting with Our Spiritual
  Intelligence*, Bloomsbury 2000
  *A scientific and philosophical presentation of the invaluable
  role of a spiritual perspective.*
Zukav, Gary, *The Seat of the Soul*, Fireside 1990
  The where, what, how and why of the soul.

AUDIOCASSETTE

The Chakra System. Spiritual Instruction with Walter Makichen.
  Centre for Self Teaching, 4001 60th St, Sacramento, CA 95820,
  Tel (916) 455-8387.
  *This outstanding series of seven lectures familiarises us with
  the personality of each chakra. They introduce us to energetic
  exercises, visualisations, and sounds that harmonise and
  evolve the chakra system.*

* *Authors' note*

INDEX

THE AUTHORS MAY BE CONTACTED AT

INSTITUTE OF PSYCHOSOCIAL MEDICINE
2 EDEN PARK, SUMMERHILL ROAD
DUN LAOGHAIRE, CO. DUBLIN
FAX (01) 284 3028
EMAIL IPMED@EIRCOM.NET